The Hearts of Men

Chris Barker has been a teacher and researcher for over 25 years and has worked in schools and universities in both England and Australia. He is currently Associate Professor of Cultural Studies at the University of Wollongong, New South Wales. Chris is the author of six previous books that are linked together by an interest in culture, meaning and communication. At present he is exploring questions of emotion and spirituality in contemporary life.

The Hearts of Men
Tales of Happiness and Despair

CHRIS BARKER

To Freya with love

A UNSW Press book
Published by
University of New South Wales Press Ltd
University of New South Wales
Sydney NSW 2052
AUSTRALIA
www.unswpress.com.au

© Chris Barker 2007
First published 2007

This book is copyright. Apart from any fair dealing for the purpose of private study, research, criticism or review, as permitted under the Copyright Act, no part may be reproduced by any process without written permission. Inquiries should be addressed to the publisher.

National Library of Australia
Cataloguing-in-Publication entry

> Barker, Chris, 1955– .
> The hearts of men: tales of happiness and despair.
>
> ISBN 9780868409498 (pbk.).
>
> 1. Men - Australia - Interviews. 2. Men - Australia - Biography. 3. Men - Australia - Psychology. 4. Men - Australia - Conduct of life. 5. Emotions - Sex differences.
>
> 305.310994

Design Josephine Pajor-Markus
Cover design Di Quick
Cover photo Karen Mork
Printer Griffin Press

Acknowledgments
I would like to thank all the men who kindly gave of their time and energy to tell me their stories. Please note pseudonyms only are used.

Contents

1	Stories of modern men	1
2	This sporting life	22
3	Why we are talking about men now	44
4	Your mum and dad	64
5	Family foundations	82
6	Men and depression	100
7	Living on drugs and alcohol	121

8	Work, work, work	*137*
9	Men and relationships	*154*
10	Changing ourselves	*174*
11	Redemption song	*194*
	Notes	*213*

Stories of modern men

STEPHEN AND HAROLD

A week after I had spoken with him, Stephen hung himself. He was 21 years old. Later, I talked with one of his close friends, Bob. 'I stopped him doing himself in once a long time ago,' he said. 'He came up to my place and was slashing his arms up and he was drunk. We grew up together. We used to live across the road from each other when we were kids. His mates are all sitting around just dumbfounded.'

Stephen told me that he felt 'angry inside'. 'I feel angry because I didn't have a father to bring me up as a son,' he said. Anger was a repeated theme of our conversation: anger with his father, anger when he witnessed male violence, the anger that drove his assault on his stepfather and a tendency to 'snap and go off my head'. More often than not, Stephen hid his anger behind a jovial facade. 'He was basically the life of the party when there was no party,' said Bob. However, like many a party animal, Stephen was fuelled by alcohol. 'He had been drinking for a long time, I know that,' continued Bob. 'He wanted to do something about it, I know, but the grog had a grip on him like nothing else.'

Stephen thought himself an alcoholic and, despite undergoing alcohol and anger management courses (ordered by courts following theft and assault convictions), he had not been able to stop drinking. Alcohol and marijuana helped to reduce his feelings of edginess, he explained – feelings[1] that had underpinned his experience of 'always getting into trouble at school'. Stephen's family had already modelled to him the value of alcohol as a 'solution' to life's difficulties. His father 'had a drinking problem' and 'he got aggressive when he was drinking with my mum and beat her around and stuff'. Eventually, Stephen's mother left the family home, taking her son with her. Stephen rarely saw his father again: 'He showed me that he had very little time for me. He only had time for his drink.'

'It's the things that affect me powerfully, emotionally, that are important to me,' said 75-year-old Harold. 'I want to go on living. I don't want it to end now because I am having such a good time.' In particular, his life as a carpenter had provided him with a sense of purpose and joy: 'Making things has been a real satisfaction for me and it has been all that I have needed throughout my life. I loved the feel of the wood and the sense of being totally absorbed in what I was doing. It made me feel good and I think everyone has to feel that they are worth something.'

Harold talked warmly and positively about his parents. 'I have good recollections of Dad. We used to go fishing together and it was a pretty good father and son team there,' he said. However, like many men, he was closer to his mother: 'I was more involved with her and I felt loved by her. It's apparent now in my mind that she was the one who imparted whatever codes of conduct that have stuck with me now.' Harold valued self-discipline, a job well done, friendships and the ethic of 'do unto others as you would be done by'.

Harold's life had not been without hardship. He had endured wartime service and suffered loss when his marriages were ended by divorce and death. Yet, Harold was resilient in the face of difficulty and accepted the circumstances of his life: 'Given the environment that I grew up in, I don't see how I could have done anything differently and

Stories of modern men

not made mistakes along the way. You could say I was happy, content. It's hardly the right word, is it? Except that everything I have done is okay.' He was even ready to face death. He was not looking forward to it, but neither was he frightened: 'I am prepared for simply going out of existence.'

MEN AND EMOTION

Stephen and Harold are talking about their emotional lives — and they are men. What a surprise! After all, there is a widespread perception that men can't express their emotions. If we were to believe everything we read in magazines or see on TV, men are tongue-tied emotional voids: empty of feeling and lacking in words, we are hardly human — and certainly deficient. But this is not so. Men are human beings; we have emotional lives and we can talk about them.

In this book, we will encounter men talking about fear, anger, love, joy, sadness, hope, happiness and despair. We will hear accounts of the complex 'hidden' emotional lives of men. These tales are hidden in the sense that we rarely hear about the emotional lives of men because our culture has discouraged us from talking about them in public. Men will often not initiate a conversation about their emotions and can be reluctant to talk about their feelings unless the conditions are right. But this does not mean that we cannot talk about emotions at all. Shakespeare was a man. Wordsworth was a man. Freud was a man!

A family I know were in the midst of a domestic crisis. The father talked to his wife about his concerns. The son was able to talk to his mother. But the father and the son remained closed-lipped together. Fathers and sons do seem to have a particularly hard time talking with each other. However, this does not mean that men *can't* talk about their emotional lives, full stop. It all depends on the context.

It is clear, nonetheless, that Stephen is from Saturn and Harold is from Jupiter, so to speak. The conditions of their lives and their emotional responses are so radically divergent. But what is it about their social circumstances and personal psychology that made Stephen despairing and Harold resilient? How shall we understand the epidemic of depression among modern men? And what is happening to men's emotional engagement with women? It is these and related questions that we tackle in this book.

What is at stake is not whether men experience emotion in their lives – they do. Nor is the central question about whether we can express feelings. The stories in this book challenge the widespread view that men cannot talk about their emotions. Rather, the significant issue concerns the *quality* of those lives and the wisdom of men's emotional communication. We will be concerned with the life circumstances and psychological strategies that give rise to happiness or despair rather more than if men experience these states. We will enquire about the skilfulness of emotional expression that men employ rather than whether men express emotion at all.

The theme of emotions and their skilful management is a major concern of our times. Emotions have always been important to us because they are central to what makes us human. However, they are emerging as a particularly visible theme of contemporary Western culture. We talk about emotions in TV chat shows, we read about emotions in magazines and we seek guidance about emotions from an array of therapists. In particular, men and their emotions are under the microscope of public scrutiny. There is a good deal of popular discussion about the behaviour of men like Stephen. From naughty boys in the schoolyard to bad – or sad – men in the public domain, men are increasingly viewed as a 'problem'.

In this book, we explore happiness and despair, joy and anguish, love and anger, success and failure in the lives of the men that I talked with. And since I am inevitably bound up in the process of telling these stories, it is also partly about myself.

In the beginning

I recall sitting in a pub at the age of 18 with two friends discussing the kind of life we wanted to live. My closest friend expressed a preference for a steady life marked by peace and calm. His girlfriend and I agreed that we would rather embrace the peaks of excitement, even if that also meant living with the lows. This proved to be a prophetic moment, or perhaps a reflection of temperament, for it was in the midst of a prolonged emotional trough that I conceived of exploring the emotional lives of men. I was already reading books about depression, but decided that I might learn by talking to other men.

Once I had embarked upon this strategy, I found that talking was therapeutic for me, as well as being an exercise in collecting stories. I discovered that many men were replicating my own encounter with depression. Consequently, 'the blues' is a subtheme of the book, not only because of my personal experience, but also because it was raised again and again by other men. Nonetheless, while a significant purpose of the book is to explore men's accounts of sadness and despair, it is also to map the pathways to greater happiness and contentment.

REMEMBERING MY FATHER

There was a particular man who prompted this investigation – my father. In recent times, I have recovered some warmer memories of him. I remember as a small boy we watched the local village hall burn down from the bottom of our garden. Many years later, I can still recall the soft touch of his cheek against mine as he held me up to see the dancing flames. I remember going with him to watch my first professional football game on my tenth birthday. I can still evoke the colour and noise of the crowd, the magical appearance of sporting heroes and his protective presence by my side. And I remember play-fighting with him on the front room floor, so often a boy's way to get cuddled by his father.

These memories have returned to me as I have come to forgiveness and put aside the anger that for many years was my predominant feeling about him. My anger was a response to his unpredictable, hostile and sometimes violent behaviour, itself a manifestation of alcoholism. Here in the family photograph album I see the black-and-white images of the man who was my father but never my dad. It's strange, he looks fragile and old and I feel sadness and loss instead of the fear and anger that was once inseparable from his simple brutish presence. I recognise the face but not the feeling. As a boy, I could smell the whiff of drunken unpredictability. I sensed the lingering threat of violence and the crackle of resentment that hung in the air like distant thunder. I could always tell when he had been drinking – and my anxiety was instantaneous.

Today, in the photograph before me I see the shadow of his fear and loneliness where once I could see only my own. As I explored the emotional lives of myself and other men, I was aware that I was also investigating him. Why was he that way, I wondered? What had made him into the monster I thought him to be? And I have found that I was not alone in this concern, since men's relationship with their fathers was a recurrent theme of my conversations. Only a small minority of adult men in Western culture can describe an emotionally stable and fulfilling connection with their father.

TO BE LOVED BY WOMEN

For heterosexual men, women are commonly at the centre of their emotional landscape. To investigate the emotional lives of men is to say something about their relationships with women. I share the wish to love and be loved by women, but have also added to the divorce statistics. I found many men who had formed long-lasting and satisfying relationships with women and I explore how this is possible. However, I also talked to men whose relationships with women have troubled them and their partners. Many of the men I spoke to reflected an age where relationships are increasingly provisional. Less 'until death do us part' and more 'until something better comes along'.

The first woman in our lives is usually our mother. I know that my mother loves me and cared for me as best she could. Her face in many a family photograph is, however, sad and disconnected. In the image before me, I am sitting on her knee smiling at her through the cracked teeth of childhood tumbles, the spark of hope still glowing in my eyes. I am a small boy with pale skinny legs that dangle down from her lap and hair that has been cut with blunted garden shears. She is dressed in fabric flowers formed by shades of dark and light that my mind transforms into red and yellow hues. She is upright and stiff, looking away into the distant nothingness. Dark of hair and eye, she is absent. Her downturned mouth suggests a woman depressed. My mother is smart, energetic, independent and brave in the face of her life's many difficulties. She loved me; but wrapped in her own pain, her love struggled to shine through.

Many of the men I talked with had happy, nurturing relationships with their mothers, although a few did not. Either way, it is clear that the emotional trajectory of our life is heavily dependent on the quality of our childhood relationships. It is useful, then, to try to understand the familial basis of one's own personality and behaviour. However, one of the most valuable lessons I learnt charting my own voyage is that it is not helpful to lay blame. Our parents had their own families of origin and personal demons to contend with. They acted out of their own conditioning, just as we do. The purpose of delving into the past is not to point the finger, but to prepare the grounds of forgiveness – for oneself and for others.

TO SEE AND TO CONQUER

Men commonly look outwards for community affirmation of their worth. In particular, they seek praise and external validation through the public world of work. I suppose the acquisition of educational qualifications and an academic writing career has been my own way of seeking this. Other men have found different routes: winning at football, managing organisations, reaching record annual profits, out-drinking their mates or being recognised for civic contributions. In any case, men's relationship with work (and its conflicts with home) is a significant theme of the book.

In the end, I am not unique among men in seeking validation through public achievement. I am not unique in having suffered from depression. I am not the only man to have been divorced and separated from his children. I am not alone in having sometimes used intoxicants. There are, as I discovered, many other men living through these kinds of experiences.

However, this is not simply a gloomy story of isolation, pain and disaster. In fact, it is rather an upbeat tale of recovery and happiness. I talked not only to men who had experienced emotional pain, but also to men who seemed to be personally, professionally and emotionally stable. I was seeking not only the root causes of the problems faced by contemporary men, but also the conditions and strategies that founded greater contentment. So, while I speak of emotional suffering, I also offer tales of hope. This is the stuff of human drama as it weaves together the emotions and life stories of its central characters.

Private lives and public stories

From soap opera to Shakespeare, drama is crafted from the emotional upheavals of our lives. We are treated to acts of kindness and acts of betrayal, the getting of wisdom and the consequences of foolishness – and with them, of course, love, anger, fear, shame, guilt and elation. Like drama, this book sets emotions within the narratives of men's lives told through multiple interwoven stories. The texture of the writing is formed by the warp and weft of a variety of tales.

First, there are the stories of over 100 men who recounted the tales of their lives in the context of loosely structured conversations.[2] The majority of these men were Anglo-Australians, though a quarter were British and American men living in Australia (and I am a migrant from England to Australia). The details of Australian men's lives are, of course, valuable in their own right. However, these life stories and emotional concerns are sufficiently similar to those of most other men in the English-speaking world to be read as a broader account of men and emotion in Anglo-Western culture.[3] As a man born in England, living in Sydney as an Australian citizen, there was nothing in the accounts of Australians and Americans that I could not understand.

Since only three of the men described themselves as gay and all but four were white, this is largely an account of white English-speaking heterosexual men in the context of Western culture. While this may appear as a limitation of the book, it also provides a level of cultural cohesion to an otherwise diverse set of stories. And it is, after all, white heterosexual men who, it is often claimed, are unable to speak about their emotions (a stark assertion this book contests).

A second strand of stories, the subplot, is made up of broader accounts of human existence that explain to us why we behave as we do. These narratives are provided by biology, psychology, philosophy, anthropology, linguistics, sociology and cultural studies. Viewing the world from these perspectives is analogous to observing the landscape through the window of a plane. We see the broad shape of things, the patterns of the human social world, but we lose a sense of proximity and detail. We may miss the fact that much of what is said about 'men' applies to some men and not to others. For this reason, I continually return to the specific details of particular men.

CULTURE AND IDENTITY

Film and television drama is concerned with the private lives of its characters, but since millions of people are watching, it is also a very public affair. Similarly, as individual men tell their specific tales they are also giving an account of a wider public culture. The apparently private, secret inner world of our emotions can be grasped as a manifestation of our collective way of life. The kinds of relationships we form and our expectations of them are shaped by our culture, which provides maps of meaning telling us who we are, where we are, and how to get from here to there. For example, as you read the brief account I gave of my parents, you will have drawn upon our shared knowledge of what mothers and fathers are expected to do. This may be quite different in another culture.

Public stories are at the heart of who we are and our ability to answer the questions: What to do? How to act? Who to be? Our personal identity is constructed from a shared language in the context of social relationships. When we read the stories of individual men, we are also investigating the way our culture understands what it is to be a man, and what we mean by emotion.

Emotions are not simply universals of biology, but are shaped by the contours of culture. When we speak about anger, fear, disgust or love, we do so as if we are referring to a distinct condition. However, if as I look you in the eye my heart is racing, my palms are sweaty and I feel a little shaky, is this fear or is it love? This depends, of course, on whether you are pointing a gun or seeking an embrace. Indeed, so much depends on the context and on what I am thinking that it is unclear that emotions are distinct states at all. Rather, anger, fear and love are names we give to experiences arising from interactions between our mind and our body and the minds and bodies of others.

Our cultural maps tell us how we should behave and how we may express emotion. For example, displays of grief in the Anglo-American world were downplayed prior to the 19th century. However, during the Victorian era grief became a culturally foregrounded emotion involving public displays and rituals. By the early 20th century, grieving was once again subject to restraint.[4] Emotions are subject to rules by which people are expected to be happy at weddings and sad at funerals (feeling rules) and to enact them in culturally approved ways (display rules). Failure to act appropriately will bring social admonishment that invokes guilt and shame (emotions implicated in social regulation). For example, businessman Peter was obliged to show emotional restraint at work after having recently fallen in love:

> I felt happier than I had been for years and I wanted to tell people about it, but it's not a good idea to show too much in business, you know. We're very task-oriented here and we're judged on what we get done. You just don't show anything that might cast a doubt over your competence. You get the job done and you keep your feelings to yourself. (Peter, aged 45)

The stories we tell about our emotional lives draw upon the scripts provided by our culture. We talk about love, family and self in ways that our shared language enables. For example, the very ideas of family trauma, a personal journey and the steps of recovery are well-established motifs of Western culture that we now deploy routinely. They are not likely to be common ways of speaking among the poor of Ethiopia or Afghanistan.

I am concerned, then, to link the broad stories of culture with the biographic details of specific lives. I hope to put living flesh on the dry skeletons of history and sociology. Indeed, biographical detail muddies the waters of grand narratives 'about men' and allows us to see their inevitable partiality. What we need to do, then, is oscillate between the big picture and the details of individual lives. The broader accounts we can read in books. The details come from speaking with living, breathing men.

Characters and conversations

Before we move more deeply into our exploration of the emotional lives of men, I would like to introduce you to some of the settings and characters in our drama. My quest began with reflections on why there are increasingly large numbers of depressed men in Western societies and why I was among them. I also wanted to understand why men like my father are so strongly implicated in alcoholism and drug addiction. I began my enquiry with a group of men who I thought might exemplify these conditions: 'at risk' homeless young people. These men all lived with forms of addiction and Stephen (above) was among their number.

DOWN AND OUT DOWN UNDER

A local newspaper article alerted me to the efforts of youth workers to assist homeless young men. The commentary highlighted the problems they faced and the part played by the drop-in centre in ameliorating their difficulties. The centre provided practical services such as breakfast and a shower as well as health advice and liaison with welfare agencies. Assisted by a youth worker, I arranged to talk with a number of the young men who used the building and the support it offered.

The 25 volunteers were mostly talkative and wanted a chance to tell their stories. Indeed, I often felt that I was acting as an unqualified counsellor by simply listening. I wanted to talk to these homeless drug users because male substance abuse, criminal behaviour, domestic violence and public disorder are front-page news. Since none of us wishes to be robbed, assaulted or intimidated, there is a tendency to demonise such men. Homeless young criminals have been the subjects of a 'moral panic'[5] by which official agencies and the media identify them as a coherent group, labelling their behaviour as troublesome and likely to reoccur. Drug users, in particular, have been characterised as contemporary 'folk devils' that must be tracked down and punished.

Yet, apparently 'bad' men often turn out to be 'sad men', the damaged goods of modern industrial society. Men's violence, sex addiction, gambling and drug abuse can be understood as self-medication that acts as a defence against covert depression.[6] Twenty-three-year-old Ben told me: 'I hate life, I hate the world. Heroin is my antidepressant' (see chapter 6). In talking to these young men, I wondered whether it was possible to comprehend and humanise the devil. As Jake unfolded his story, I began to think that it was. Jake was born in New Zealand, but came to Australia as a baby. He was 23 years old at the time of our conversation.

Jake's story[7]

My dad got divorced when I was two and I had a stepdad who abused me physically and emotionally. My real dad – I don't know where he is. I copped all of the abuse from my stepdad because he didn't like me. I was in foster care so many times before I was 12 and Mum was in a women's refuge. My mum kicked me out when I was 16 and I've been out of home ever since; that was seven years ago. But I don't want to blame anyone; I just want to let go of the past and move on.

I got depressed at 17 and then I was diagnosed with having schizophrenia and a nervous disorder and severe depression and I've been going in and out of hospital ever since. I get suicidal. When I'm very depressed I don't eat, I don't do anything; I stay inside in my bed. I take it out on myself. I look in the mirror and I'll smash the mirror or I'll do something nasty to myself. I think about hanging myself. I put a rope around my neck. I was just sitting there on a branch with a rope around my neck and all I wanted to do was stand up on the branch and just fall down and let my neck crack.

I was brought up in a place where they dealt in drugs. Nothing beat the feeling at the time when I was using heroin. It just numbs you, it comfortably numbs you. You can just sit back and relax and nothing will bother you. But it was a habit that was too expensive to keep going. I got into crime. I got into break and entering, getting caught by the police, and all of a sudden I just said 'That's it, I've had enough'. I just went cold turkey. It was hard, the muscle cramps were coming and I was spewing and the constipation was happening and I was losing a lot of weight.

I found a girlfriend and settled down. We didn't plan for a baby, but the baby came so I stuck by her anyway. She's pregnant again; she's due in November. She's a beautiful girl, but she suffers from a mental illness as well and she can't take any medication because it might affect the unborn child. She's had Hepatitis C for five years or so. But I don't know how long she's gonna live for; it's hard to say. But I will stick by her and

Stories of modern men

try my best to love her. I don't want her to go, I don't want her to die; it's a sad feeling.

I picture myself in a corner crying a lot, in a dark room; that's the picture that I'm in; with my head in my hands just crying. What stops me from doing anything to harm myself is God. Or call it a Higher Power; you just sit down by the sea; you just think 'man this is a big world and who created this and what are we doing here and what's happening' and then you think of God. I still don't know what my future is, but everything is gonna be all right in the end. I'm determined, like I gave up all the drugs and the alcohol. I'm pushing myself forward like a soldier just going through the war. There's a war going inside me all the time; it's good and bad; they're always fighting.

The tales that Jake and his friends told me gave me an insight into their world. However, in order to grasp the self-destructive aspects of some men's emotional lives, I also needed to understand those of us who seemed to be happy and successful. So I broadened the scope of my investigation to cover a variety of men from different walks of life, including the world of corporate business. These were men who exemplified socially sanctioned success in Western culture. Surely they were happy.

EXECUTIVE DRIVE

Standing at the foot of a sky-busting commercial tower of tinted glass and steel, I feel overshadowed by this phallic monument to male power and money. After checking in at the reception desk, I travel by 21st-century space-age transport to the upper echelons of corporate decision-making. The view from the top floor is truly awesome. I can see across the city and beyond to the fringes of the metropolis. I have come to interview one of 20 influential business executives whose life stories form a part of the book.

It takes an hour and a half to drive from the drop-in centre for 'at risk' young men to Telecom Tower, the headquarters of a multinational communications corporation. The journey from one interviewee to another is only 90 kilometres, but the social and emotional worlds inhabited by homeless teenagers and corporate executives are galaxies apart. Men may be from Mars and women from Venus, but the cultural distance between men can be greater. Yet, love and hope, anger and despair are significant emotions in both these universes. The public gulf is vast, but there remains a bridge of common human feelings. We all suffer, we all have the potential to experience joy and we all need love and human connection.

The stable family backgrounds of corporate executives are in striking contrast to the chaotic and emotionally painful childhoods of heroin users. However, these task-oriented and success-driven executives struggled to find a balance between their emotional connections and the demands of working life. For example, Gerard was a senior manager with a multinational telecommunications corporation. He was born in the United Kingdom and came to Australia when he was two years old. He was 36 at the time of the interview.

Gerard's story

I guess the jobs I've done for the last few years have been stressful, but some of the opportunities that are associated with that are absolutely fascinating. The economic rewards are very generous. I suppose typically I would start some time between seven-thirty and eight and in a usual day I'd probably finish between seven and eight. I'd probably do a few hours on the weekend, depending upon how busy the week coming up is. So the hours are reasonably long.

The greatest difficulty that I have is that I'm single and I live by myself. It means there's nobody saying you've got to get home by this particular time, so often the easiest thing to do is just keep working. You can find yourself getting into patterns where you're working and not doing a whole lot else and then you have to kind of try and arrest that. So trying to make regular arrangements to meet up with friends is important: not always easy, because many of my friends have jobs with similar demands on them.

A lot of domestic service I buy in, I have a cleaner and so on, and the lifestyle I lead is quite a selfish one. On the other hand, you know, I've chosen to live alone, so when I go home, my house is dark and there's nobody there and so I spend a lot of time by myself when I'm not working. So that's a negative; but you know, one makes these trade-offs.

My mother was always somebody who I could go to and say I have a problem with this or that or whatever. My relationship with my father was strained for much of my adolescence and I guess early to mid-twenties. As I look back, I see that my father allocated a lot of time to me. He spent a lot of time coaching me to get a scholarship. Over the last few years, our relationship has improved greatly now that we have shared professional interests; that gives us a connection that we perhaps didn't have a few years ago.

As a child, I think you see the messages that your parents send through their behaviour. The model I saw my parents set was one of steady, solid work and it was a house with lots of books and so on. I did very well academically at school. It was clear that I was going to university; the question was Law or Medicine, you know, it was that simple. And at about the age of 15 I decided it was Law and I didn't think about it again.

Gerard's concern, as an unmarried man, was how to work long hours, maintain contact with friends and meet someone with whom he could conduct a sexual relationship. For most of the other executives, the central problem lay in deflecting the considerable criticism they faced from wives and children about the long hours they spent at work. They frequently expressed regret that work so often subtracted from their personal lives. They said that they understood the need for greater emotional openness and negotiation. Nevertheless, they continued to devote most of their time to work. They were not yet willing or able to change the order of their commitments to prioritise relationships.

As James (aged 49) told me: 'I work hard and I work long hours. I want success at work and sometimes my family life suffers. I know that, that's the life I choose.' In this, they were not unlike their fathers' generation, who were trained not only in hard work but also in war, the archetypical activities of the 'disposable gender'.[8] It was to talk with these old soldiers that I now journeyed.

PUTTING UP WITH HARDSHIP

The Diggers Rest Home is situated about a kilometre inland from the main coastal road that runs south of the city. 'Digger' is a term for a member of the Australian armed forces and dates back to the First

World War. The residential home is a rather unassuming, if not to say ugly, brick building where I had arranged to talk with 25 men who had served in the army during the Second World War, or who had worked in 'protected' occupations.

The rest home is well positioned to catch the morning sun, which many of the older more frail residents take advantage of by sitting out on the veranda to chat, read or snooze. But this is no luxury retirement village for the well-heeled. The residents' rooms are cell-like and the dining room reminded me of forgotten schooldays with its parallel lines of formica-topped tables. Despite the valiant efforts of staff and residents to decorate the bare-brick walls, the place has a spartan feel to it. Money is in short supply and the residents are not harbouring large private superannuation funds or drawing outsized pensions. The home is adequate but basic, echoing in its very fabric a theme of these men's lives, the coming to terms with hardship. As 75-year-old Victor told me: 'You have got to learn how to put up with hard things. You have to have patience and endure it.' One of the particular hardships for this generation of men was the experience of war. As Edward, aged 89, said: 'I felt it was my duty to volunteer.'

Edward's story

My father was a farm labourer, bush worker, builder of houses, all sorts of things. I followed in his footsteps and wanted to be a farm labourer. He was a good dad. My mother was quite a nice lady too; we got on well together. I think I was as close as any of the family. There were 11 and after my mother died my father married again and had two more. Yes, a fairly happy family life; very poor, very needy and for that reason it was a hard life. But we lived.

At 25, I married. I met up with a lady and she was 13 years older than me and we were married for 55 years. She was a lovely wife too. We had no children, I don't know why. We could see the good things about it and we could see the bad things about it; we expected children but then we didn't have them. Things were hard in those days. So we just counted our blessings as we were. I worked on the farm for years after we married and then the war broke out when I was 28.

I enlisted in June 1941 and found myself in Singapore and around Kuala Lumpur. We were taken prisoner and we were captured and put into Changi Prison. I spent three months in Changi and then a group of us were taken by ship from Singapore up to Burma and we were set to work on the Burma Railway line. It was slave labour. It was the biggest war crime as far as we were concerned. It took ten months to build the line; quite a lot of them were killed and some were taken to Japan. We had to face up to most things and we had to take them in our stride. It's surprising what you can take if you have to.

After the war, I returned to Tasmania and when I was ready I started work on the farm and I found that I just couldn't do it. I didn't have the strength to settle down. It was not fit for a person who had been shattered. My wife was marvellous. It was our life together; we just simply started again where we left off. I just think she was a lovely girl. We both had plenty of common sense.

Anyway, I then took on this university study for a degree in Theology. So I decided to join the ministry. I was converted to Christianity at age 20. Christianity has been a help to me, it has strengthened my resolve to go and do the right things, which you don't always do. Christianity doesn't mean that you are perfect in any way. It's not failure as long as you try. You have to live with Christian values. I've had disappointments, of course, but somehow you get by. Happiness is not the word. Contented is more the word. I would say that I have lived a contented life believing in Jesus Christ.

This generation of men suffered hardship while simultaneously being trained not to speak publicly about their feelings. To their children and grandchildren, they are the archetype of 'emotionally repressed' men. Yet, they were able and willing to speak about their emotions when asked. A stoical acceptance of life's ups and downs, which marked out the emotionally contented from those still riding the roller-coaster of human feelings, should not be confused with an *inability* to express emotion.

For Edward, this equanimity was a by-product of his Christian convictions, and while this quality can be developed in other ways, it is often a feature of 'spirituality'. I talked to two groups of men who have sought solutions to life's difficulties through philosophies that have a 'spiritual' dimension – one ancient and one modern.

PATHS TO HAPPINESS

The recent growth of the 'men's movement' and Buddhism in Western culture (Buddhism has a 2500-year-old history in Asia) can be understood through their links with 'self-help' culture. Neither Buddhism nor the men's movement are forms of clinical psychology, but they share a concern for emotional wellbeing. In particular, they focus on the skilful management of difficult emotions and the cultivation of happiness or contentment.

At its worst, the men's movement (which is not homogeneous) blames women for men's problems. However, at its best it furthers self-reflection and emotional intelligence. The men I talked with cut across any ideological divisions. They supported justice for women, but also identified the distinctive characteristics of men. They were more concerned with self-analysis, consciousness-raising and personal change than with adversarial political campaigning. These interviewees were concerned with emotions and relationships because they felt that changes in men's personal behaviour would initiate changes in the wider culture.

During my experience of depression, I turned to Western psychology, of course, but was also attracted to the connections between Buddhism and psychotherapy: an East–West dialogue in the time of globalisation. Buddhism stresses the need for self-awareness through the practices of meditation and mindfulness. Charles is a 50-year-old Australian and former monk turned lay Buddhist teacher who practises continual self-reflection and growth. As he told me: 'The one true path is awareness and love and compassion and nobody has a monopoly on them. It's something you work on; it's a process. It's always a process; there's always something you need to work on.'

Charles's story

My relationship with my father was distant and it became troublesome when I was in my late teens. It was clear from his point of view that I was pretty useless, like I wasn't coping with anything. He was an alcoholic; he was a jovial drunk. I come from a long line of male alcoholics. I became very angry with him.

Originally, the Church defined my universe, what the world was, was what the Church said the world was. I decided that I really wanted to be a priest. That place was the first time I really felt at home. The first year was really good, but the second year was getting difficult. I was 16 and I got into a crisis, which made it impossible for me to continue. God had disappeared, so there was a void, but this void was real and it was incredibly powerful. I was in this black, utterly alone, total aloneness and it would be like that forever. I lost faith in conventional Christianity. I couldn't believe the things that you were supposed to believe; because I knew that doctrines were just doctrines, they're not the reality.

I was deeply depressed, basically, until I discovered meditation. When I discovered Buddhism, I thought I have to do this. I went to Hawaii [Zen Meditation Centre] to do the summer training, but ended up staying two years. I'm still inclined to a certain sorrowful nature, but those severe depressions were gone. Then in '84 I went to Burma for the first time and I met X and really connected with what he was teaching. This was much more skilful and sophisticated than anything I had done before. I did a three-month retreat and that was a major turning point.

There has always been some part of me that has wanted to settle down with a companionable woman and have a domestic scene. I would have liked a long-term partner to share what I was doing. But if I had to choose between the path that I was on and a relationship, I would choose the path; that was always more important. And even today in reality that's the case. So in a sense I accept loneliness as part of the price that has to be paid. Maybe what I'm going through is the legacy of a family who didn't communicate very skilfully and I'm going to have to learn new habits.

A spiritual life is a life that isn't based on simply gaining material possessions or position; that goes deeper than that. From what I've seen of family life, I think family life is a spiritual life because people are devoted to each other and forego any material gain. That to me is a spiritual life, one that has a deeper aspect of creating a mental happiness and contentment. It's not dependent on material circumstances.

Somewhat surprisingly, Charles was a surreptitious fan of rugby league. After all, a group of big blokes crashing into each other chasing an oval ball is in stark contrast to the serenity associated with Buddhism. Spirituality is not a frequent topic on *The Footy Show*, and sportsmen have often been perceived as 'men behaving badly', with alcohol abuse and sexual misconduct featuring prominently. However, the discussions

I had with sportsmen were the ones that surprised me the most because they did not conform to that stereotype. On the contrary, they were mainly more balanced and emotionally secure than the other men I spoke with.

THE GAME OF LIFE

Sport plays an important part in our culture and the prominent place it holds in men's lives makes it a valuable site to explore attitudes and emotions. Throughout this book, I shall be drawing on conversations with 20 men for whom sport was at the heart of their lives. Half of these men were full-time professional sportsmen[9], while the remainder were semi-professionals and 'dedicated amateurs'.[10]

All of these men are 'successful' sportsmen because they play at an elite level. That they are skilful is significant because I want to explore the attitudes and emotional strategies that contribute to sporting achievement. These include the will and discipline to improve one's performance. As Craig, aged 30 and a professional rugby league player, told me: 'You know, whatever I did I always wanted to be the best at it. The best I could be.' For Alex, a 23-year-old professional rugby union player, a similar philosophy takes on an almost spiritual cast: 'I've had a couple of friends who have died when they were reasonably young and I think the one thing that I gained massively out of their deaths is that it's a finite period of time that you have. Every single day you get up, you've got to do it like it was your last.'

Alex's story

I was really good at sport, which is an easy way to get friends and relationships set up. In that regard, you know, I fitted in pretty well. We lived close to the beach and I surfed all the time and so we had really good mates around the area. It probably kept us out of a lot of trouble because at that age, trouble usually results from boredom. Every spare minute we'd have, we'd be at the beach doing something.

Rugby was like the cornerstone on which we based our school around; rugby was everything. Like, we were the best school purely based on the fact that we won the rugby competition every year. Even now, like, the guys that I see from school, because I play for the X and stuff, they'd look at that as a really big thing and I do this for a living now.

Mum and Dad, like, because they were really high achievers at school and I was the first child, they really expected me to be like them and they thought, 'Gee, he's good at sport, but that's not that important'. When I got my High School Certificate back, Mum asked me if I was gonna be a furniture removalist, you know, she was horrified and she couldn't believe that I had done so badly.

I never thought I'd actually play at a professional level. So how far can I go? I just say to myself, 'Look, do the best you can, train as hard as you can, do as well as you can, because the rest will take care of itself'. You can't do anything more than that and if I don't make it and I've done my best, well then I'm happy with what I've done.

I don't put any time into negative thoughts because it's not gonna help me, it will only make me feel bad. Maybe a quarter of 1 per cent of my life would be focused on the glass is half empty or something negative and I'll always try and turn it around to a positive. I've just said to myself, 'If I can control it, then why would I want to feel bad and why would I want to feel negative, when, as long as I make things positive I'll always have a positive outcome?'. It's all about just living and doing the best you can at the time you're doing it and knowing at the end of the day that if tomorrow was your last that you've done everything you could.

Football codes have a reputation for alcohol abuse and sexual misconduct. Certainly, drinking lies at the heart of their social activity. However, I found less evidence of alcohol and drug abuse among these particular sportsmen than among other men. I also found less evidence of depression. These sportsmen were the least emotionally distressed group with whom I spoke. This was highly unexpected. Because the public face of sport often seems to exemplify men's emotional troubles, I had in fact targeted them as a likely trouble spot. I was wrong. Indeed, as we shall see in our next chapter, these particular sportsmen exemplified some attitudes and behaviours that are promoted by Western psychology (and Buddhism) as the foundations of happiness.

This sporting life

Men have long been associated with sport: playing it, watching it and talking about it. Of course, sport is important to many women also, but I am concerned here with its place in the lives of boys and men. Sport plays a significant part in our cultural life, where it receives colossal media coverage and offers considerable financial rewards, mainly to men. Yet, while television applauds the 'extraordinary' talents of sporting stars, ordinary boys and men play it day in, day out on street corners and in local parks. For elderly men from the rest home, sport was an arena for developing 'friendships, football team-mates, things like that' (Max, aged 87) and constituted one of the main ways they interacted with their fathers.

The popularity that came with captaining the school cricket team meant that for 48-year-old Tony, a chief executive officer, 'high school was a very pleasant experience'. Indeed, many of the businessmen told me that sport was a good way to fit in at school. For a few like Graham (aged 48), sport entailed high-level achievement, including state and national representative honours. It was valued because it gave you 'a sense of fitness, camaraderie, success, achievement and belonging'. He saw these characteristics as an important preparation for the business world. For Derek, sport was simply an enjoyable physical activity that allowed him to 'express a bit more aggression. For me, sport was one way of how I did express myself in a more masculine way because I see myself as being a more softer person' (Derek, aged 49).

I enjoy watching sport and as a boy I enjoyed playing sport. I also get pleasure from exercise, which includes running, walking and swimming. I occasionally watch rugby league (for my sins, I follow the Sydney Roosters) and, above all, I get a great deal of satisfaction from football (I'm a lifelong fan of Tottenham Hotspur in the English Premier League). However, I did hate being *made* to do cross-country running at school and I do recognise that not all men like to play or watch games. Some men understandably view sport as an oppressive place of intimidation and bullying. Nevertheless, the prominent place that sport holds in many men's lives makes it is a useful vantage point to explore their attitudes and feelings. Sport is nothing if not an emotional experience for players and spectators alike. However, at first glance the view is not always uplifting, given the reputation that sportsmen have as 'men behaving badly'.

SHAME AND SURPRISE

The sporting hall of shame includes Australian cricket captain Ricky Ponting's 1999 drunken brawl in a Sydney pub, which highlighted his self-confessed drinking problem. While Ponting has resurrected himself, his former team-mate Shane Warne was banned for breaches of cricket's drug codes and gained a worldwide reputation for sleazy mobile phone text messages and allegations of sexual harassment. A series of incidents have been reported involving Australian rugby league players in alcohol-fuelled acts of violence or alleged sexual assault. The most high-profile incidents involved players from the Canterbury Bulldogs in allegations of sexual assault and various members of the New South Wales State of Origin team sent home following curfew-busting drinking sessions.

In England, football has thrown up a number of players with well-publicised drinking problems, including former Arsenal and England player Tony Adams (who served a jail sentence for drink-driving), Tottenham star Paul Gasgoine, whose career was stunted by his alcoholism, and perhaps most famously George Best, who eventually lost his life to alcohol-induced liver failure. Things are no better in the United States, where college football teams have a reputation for drinking, violence and sexual intimidation. Boxer Mike Tyson is a convicted rapist and leading American basketball star Koby Bryant was charged with a similar offence (the case was dismissed, but the married star admitted to having sex with his 19-year-old accuser).

Professional sportsmen have a public reputation for alcohol abuse and excessively macho, undisciplined behaviour. What a surprise, then, that the sportsmen I spoke to did not conform to that stereotype. On the contrary, they were among the more emotionally secure and least distressed group of men I talked with. They had the lowest incidence of depression, minimal alcohol abuse and were the men emotionally the closest to their fathers.

This reflects, I suggest, their purposeful and self-disciplined attitudes of mind, the antidepressant qualities of physical activity and the emotional solidity that comes from being connected to a strong social network. In fact, the attributes of emotionally contented sportsmen prefigure those we shall later encounter in relation to 'spirituality' and the positive psychology of happiness.

In this chapter, I concentrate on men for whom playing sport currently forms a central part of life. I draw on discussions with 20 men who were either full-time professional sportsmen or 'dedicated amateurs' (see chapter 1 for details). That they are committed and enthusiastic is significant because we are exploring the attitudes, attributes and emotional strategies required for achievement in sport, and their extension into life more generally. Significantly, accomplishment in sport is not simply a matter of physical attributes and capabilities but also of mental attitude and emotional intelligence.

It's a mind game

From professional golf to rugby league, the sportsmen I talked with stressed the importance of the way one *thinks* to their success. Psychologists refer to this as *cognitive processes*. For example, professional golfer Damian told me that 'it's 80 per cent mental, this game, and 20 per cent physical capability', while rugby league stalwart Craig suggested that 'you have to be hard on yourself mentally even to do the training'. Above all, I was told, a purposeful and constructive outlook is required to achieve success.

JEFF: AN OPTIMISTIC OUTLOOK

Jeff (aged 44) was a former British Olympic athlete and medal winner turned elite-level coach. His goal, he said, was to get sportsmen into a positive routine of good habits in order for them to achieve the best of which they are capable. He aimed to develop commitment, optimism, self-discipline and the drive to self-satisfaction through achievement. As a coach, Jeff tried to instil in his athletes the confident and hopeful philosophy of 'Have a go, McEnroe. Have a bloody go, son. Have a shot. If you have a go, you never know. And if you have a go, you have tried your best.' He told me that the relationship between sport and everyday life is a two-way street: a constructive outlook is needed to achieve in sport, but also, participation in sport can develop day-to-day confidence and self-control.

> Sport has taught me about application and the fact that application will be rewarded. I think sport teaches you a tremendous amount about yourself and how to achieve things. So that the discipline that sport imposed on me has definitely flown through. Everything I have achieved has been through application and hard work. (Jeff, aged 44)

Rob (aged 40) had considerable experience recruiting and training young players for a high-profile state team that feeds into the Australian international rugby side. He suggested that in any given national schoolboy cohort there would be 60-plus youngsters of roughly equal skill. Twenty-five of these young men would participate in their youth high performance program; of which only about four or five would reach the elite level. The difference between those who achieve international recognition and those who do not 'is largely mental; a lot has to do with the personality type of the person who makes it,' he said.

> The really determined ones will pick up the advice and the ball and they will run with it and they will improve their skills and improve the quality of their performance. They'll want feedback and they will want to know

X and Y; there'll be progress. The ones who aren't going to make it are the ones who go 'Oh, yeah yeah, I'll kick on without your support'. (Rob, aged 40)

SPORTING PSYCHOLOGY

Similarly, Martin, a basketball coach, articulated his philosophy of the sporting life as 'Do the best you can, be the best you can', a widely articulated viewpoint among sportsmen. Indeed, the importance of having the 'right attitude' is now a maxim of sports psychology. Our sporting 'common sense' suggests that we need to 'be positive', 'look on the bright side', 'get on with life', 'develop good habits', and so forth.

This popular wisdom is built up over time by incorporating into sporting cultures aspects of more formal philosophies. There is an 'interactive loop' between common sense and formal psychology by which each helps to constitute the other. The theme of 'positive thinking' is generated by psychologists and taken up again by coaches and players, who are then studied by psychologists. The whole complex of attitudes, values, identities and emotions in professional sport is a circular process in which the men are both the players and the played.

> I read a book on sports psychology and it basically said 'Look, you're in charge of your own thoughts and whatever you think is how your life will be' ... I don't put any time into negative thoughts because it's not going to help me. Even in death, like people that have died that are close to me, I've reflected about it and I ask myself 'How can this improve my life?' and 'How can this make me better?' It's a whole battle of keeping that mental thing positive and that's probably one of the biggest things for sportsmen. (Alex, aged 23, professional rugby player)

The cognitive aspects of sport are significant because there is a great deal of research to suggest that constructive, optimistic and hopeful thoughts generate more emotionally contented states. The centrality of 'positive' thoughts to emotion and performance is a core proposition of psychological research into depression and happiness. In particular, a sense of meaning and purpose is at the heart of joyfulness.

TIM: A SENSE OF PURPOSE

For these men, playing sport was closely associated with the notion of challenging oneself, which in turn gave them a sense of purpose and determination.

> I enjoy the challenge of the physical and the mental sort of thing. Being able to push yourself. I like the feeling of knowing that you are working hard. Knowing that you have won something is really good, but even more than that, just knowing that you have fought hard with somebody. (Tim, aged 22, Australian Football League player)

A 'challenge' entails pressing oneself towards a personal best performance. This gives sportsmen a sense of meaning, purpose and direction. Tom (aged 38: hockey) told me that 'most of my motivation has been about competing to the best of my ability'. Rick (aged 30: AFL) wanted to 'be the best that I can' and Ashley (aged 23: rugby) 'liked being the best and that drove me on'. For Rob (rugby coach, aged 40), 'being the best that you can is important. I couldn't stand playing second grade. I can't stand being second best'. To achieve our best requires motivation, drive and determination, as Craig suggests:

> You know, whatever I did I always wanted to be the best at it. The best I could be. So if there was a reason why I couldn't be the best at it, I'd go away and work at it and practise at it until I was. (Craig, aged 30, professional rugby league player)

On the face of it, seeking 'a challenge' or 'being the best' is an individualistic outlook that dovetails with sportsmen's repeated commitment to competitiveness. However, this individual search for achievement, which is simultaneously the pursuit of purpose, takes place within the context of family, friends and team-mates. In other words, sport is a complex social activity.

It's a team game

Craig grew up with a group of 'mates' with whom he played sport, especially cricket and rugby league, since the age of five. Playing games 'just happened because it was part of family life'. Sport was intrinsic to his social life and a medium for forging emotional bonds with other people. Indeed, a repeated motif of my conversations with players and coaches was that 'this is a team game'. Craig told me that rugby league players are all expected to contribute to camaraderie and, while you get the 'odd wanker', 'they don't last too long' unless they are performing exceptionally well on the pitch.

One might take exception to the idea that participating in a sporting team involves pressure on its members to conform. However, this is true of all kinds of social and cultural groups. Churches and chess clubs also expect their members to behave in particular kinds of ways. Of course, some men feel that a particularly authoritarian, macho form of discipline arises in sport and this is a question to which we shall return. For the time being, I want to acknowledge that sport forges connections with other people, and connecting with others is a fundamental requirement for emotional stability and happiness.

Physical games appeared in the lives of these sportsmen from an early age through play with local boys in backyards or neighbourhood sports fields. This was what 'mates' did together as they forged friendships. Indeed, the formation of social relationships and attachments often motivates men to participate in sport.

ALEX: THE ACCEPTANCE OF MY PEERS

Alex, a young rugby professional, recounted a childhood in which swimming, surfing, basketball, rugby and riding bikes brought together and sustained a network of friends. His social position within his peer group was enhanced by his sporting prowess. As a boy at primary school:

> I was really good at sport, which is an easy way to get friends and relationships set up, and in that regard, you know, I fitted in pretty well. Like, we were always out doing stuff and we were encouraged to do that. Later, at boarding school I fitted in well. I did rowing and rugby and I made the first teams straight away and I got the acceptance of my peers very quickly. (Alex, aged 23)

Attaining the acceptance of his peers was important for Alex: like all of us, he wanted to be recognised and valued within his social network. When we are valued by others, we develop a sense of self-worth and with it, paradoxically, the capacity for autonomous action. By contrast, depression and anxiety are associated with isolation and social insecurity. It is no coincidence that games are a social activity and that sportsmen indicated low incidence of depression.

Coaches understand social activity to be part of players 'bonding' as a team and encourage sportsmen to spend time together. 'There is a big ethos around getting together as a group of guys. You know there will be 70 or 80 guys from the football team, all drinking, and they'll be drunk by the end of it, watching this test, and that's the whole culture of rugby,' said Alex. Of course, when drinking is at the core of male friendships it comes with built-in dangers. Nonetheless, the social aspects of sporting teams can also provide the basis for self-esteem.

MITCH AND WILLIAM: GAINING RESPECT

Mitch, an international cricketer, grew up watching his two sporting brothers and observed that 'they were held in esteem by the community so that it seemed that was the way to get respect'. When he found that he was good at football and cricket: 'That boosted me straight away in life and I found that if I worked at it I got better and I became pretty good ... and I gained respect amongst the family' (Mitch, aged 35). As he commented, 'success breeds success'. Indeed, all the sportsmen confirmed that being skilful at sport was a way for them to gain admiration and popularity at school.

William (aged 30), an athlete, found his self-esteem growing with his prowess at running: 'It's good to have something you're good at and keep being good at it.' Like other sportsmen, the praise he received for his accomplishments from significant adults was important. He told me how as a young man he was fortunate to meet 'the person that inspires, drives and initiates. The move for me was my school teacher, he opened a Pandora's box'. William's teacher provided the commendation and motivation that was subsequently built on by a professional athletics coach. (However, as we shall see in chapter 6, there is a link between 'failure' and depression for William.)

Sport is a multifaceted and shared endeavour involving family and friends. For Martin (aged 40), the esteem he received from being a professional basketball coach was more important to him than wealth. Martin's income would have been greater as an accountant, but sport gave him a greater sense of purpose and esteem. The recognition of family and friends that he had achieved something to be proud of was particularly important to him. Indeed, it is significant that these sportsmen mostly told me about stable, loving family backgrounds. As we shall see later, this forms a stark contrast to the sense of abandonment felt by depressed young drug users who had experienced more emotionally chaotic childhoods.

It's a family game

Jeff, a former Olympic athlete and medallist, told me about his mother:

> She was madly in love with me and I was madly in love with her. Whatever it took in those days, she did for me and I saw that. Tremendous love by my mother. Loved by my father, but I didn't accept it in the same way that I accepted love from my mother'. (Jeff, aged 44)

With the odd exception, these successful sportsmen hailed from stable supportive families. Only one man's parents had divorced and he remained close with them both. Unsurprisingly, mothers provided the bulk of the overt emotional support and intimacy they received as children. Louis, the professional basketball player who described his mother as 'fairly cool with me my whole life', was unusual.

Rugby coach Rob (aged 40) was one of the lucky ones: he felt loved by both his parents. He described his relationship with his mother as strong – 'Mum was great' – and that with his father, to whom he felt close, as good. His father had also been a professional 'player of note', who 'would have seen all the matches I ever played in'. Likewise, Rick (aged 30), a dedicated amateur Australian Rules football player/coach and professional physiotherapist, told of 'very supportive parents' and 'a very stable family background'. He continued to feel close to his sports-loving father: 'Dad's pretty much like me in that he loves his sport, so I went and watched him play cricket and played cricket with him and I still play golf with him … we have always done stuff like that together.'

CRAIG: A GREAT RELATIONSHIP

Craig played professional rugby league in Australia for many years, representing both his state and his country.

> I think I've got a great relationship with both my parents. When I was younger, I probably had a better relationship with my mum, only because I spent more time with her, I suppose. Dad was always involved in football, rugby league, and when I was younger Dad had his own business … so he used to start very early … But you know, I love my dad very much and I think the same goes the other way around. We are a very close family. You know, it is not until you look back, you know when you are a kid you think that it's normal whatever your life is and it's not until you look back that I think, you know, I wish Dad would have spent more time with me. (Craig, aged 30)

Craig's family life offers important insights into the emotional lives of sportsmen. First, a supportive home environment can play a significant part in sporting prowess. As he explained, professional rugby is a demanding life and young men need emotional backup to sustain mental focus. Friends or a respected coach might play this role, but 'it helps if they come from a good family'. Second, Craig felt emotionally closer to his father than do many sons because of shared sporting interests. Indeed, fathers who participate in sport often encourage their sons to play games. Third, despite his solid relationship with his father and their shared love of sport, Craig still wished they had spent more time together.

Craig captures the general tenor of sportsmen's attitudes towards their families of origin. They talked about being loved, but felt more emotionally connected as children to their mothers than their fathers. This was the case despite the connection of joint male sporting activity, which was the case for three-quarters of these men.

> Dad loved me and things. Drove me to school and that sort of thing. Every night, he'd come home and we'd go down to the nets and have a hit, that sort of thing. But it wasn't one of those deep emotional we-talk-about-our-feelings kind of a relationship. (Craig, aged 30)

A 'supportive' and 'active' male parent does not always translate into an immediate verbally expressive emotional intimacy between father and son. Fathers were often practically supportive without being overtly warm. Five of the 20 sportsmen described their relationship with their fathers as 'close and loving', but the remainder felt them to be somewhat emotionally 'distant'.

Nonetheless, joint sporting activity did lead more sportsmen into active relationships with their fathers than I found among other men. A number of the sportsmen commented that their relationship with their fathers had grown closer as they got older. As young boys, they looked to their mothers for emotional proximity while simultaneously developing a more action-oriented relationship with their fathers that, if they were fortunate, laid the foundations for future intimacy. In other words, the style and trajectory of father–son intimacy diverges from that of mothers and sons.

It's a social game

TOM: CREATING A SOCIAL NETWORK

For some men the peer pressures surrounding sport are a nightmare, but for many others it is through games that they forge the emotional bonds of friendship. These collective aspects of sport extend beyond the playing field into social clubs where women and non-team members participate. Tom, the 38-year-old president (and player-coach) of a prestigious non-professional men's hockey club, told me that the value of sport to him, and to the wider community, lies in its development of social networks:

> We try hard to be a social club. You know, it's not all about study, it's not all about the pure excellence of sport, it's about developing a social network and integrating into society and that is what we are trying to do on the social side. I think that is where sport, for the majority of people, that

is the major benefit. The elite programs in place recognise that children at a young age can't sacrifice their lives to sport, they have to be fully developed and that is an acknowledgment that they are multifaceted ... the social interaction is above all the prime thing. (Tom, aged 38)

A sports club functions as a social hub through which people form all manner of emotional connections. Although Tom did have a girlfriend, he thought that we can develop an unhealthy reliance on single relationships and that it was just as important 'to get nourishment from sport or community involvement'. This includes business associations that assist players to find jobs that supplement their semi-professional income or offers them a career when pro-sport comes to an end.

DRINKING TOGETHER

Alcohol consumption is commonly associated with the social dimension of a sporting life and, undoubtedly, some sportsmen abuse alcohol. Male team sports, in particular, have a reputation for a drinking culture. As Rick (aged 30) explained: 'It's a part of sport and all the sports I've played, team sports, ever since I was 18, you finish a game and have a beer, you know, that's what you do.' Rob (aged 40) confirmed that in rugby 'alcohol is part and parcel of the whole gig'. The corporate boxes at big games involve considerable alcohol consumption, as do bars at rugby clubs for players and supporters.

Rob had played both rugby league and rugby union at elite levels and his preference was for the latter. He regarded league culture as more macho, tribal and insular, with drugs and alcohol being a greater problem than in rugby union. In league, alcohol was 'very much a part of the game and it was all beer, you know, back to the pub after training. Yes you drank a lot, too much beer'. Young rugby union professionals also told me about periods of excessive drinking, especially when they were at college. However, this had ended when a professional career became a reality. From a rugby league player came both confirmation and denial:

> I think rugby league has got that culture, you know, we train hard and we go and have a few beers together. That's part of a team sport. You know,

> I don't drink to excess, like I might have a big night or something like that, but only in a team sort of thing. I wouldn't touch a drop during the week, then I might go out and have a half-dozen beers and a few wines or something like that. (Craig, aged 30)

Rob told me that alcohol did not play a significant part in the lives of most elite rugby players in state and national teams. The coaching staff restricted access to alcohol with strict rules and strong sanctions. He named a couple of players who, over the past year, had been disciplined for drink-related activities, describing one former international player as 'shocking when he gets on the piss'. However, this was mitigated with an explanation of the player's troubled background and citing examples of current team members who did not drink at all during the season.

I had expected to hear more tales of 'sex 'n' drugs 'n' rock 'n' roll' from sportsmen than I did. Instead, most of them distanced themselves from excess alcohol and illegal drug use, describing it as incompatible with sporting achievement. For example, Brett (aged 23) had a troubled youth involving excess marijuana and alcohol, but had put this behind him when a basketball career beckoned. I was frequently told that for each sportsman who drank to excess there were two who did not drink at all. Of course, this is only a small sample and people do not always tell us the full story. Nevertheless, I formed the impression of a sporting culture in which alcohol played a significant part, but in which most men kept within the bounds of wider cultural norms.

It's a physical game

We have concentrated thus far on the highly significant social-emotional dimension of sport. However, sport also has important physical-emotional aspects. Many boys and men enjoy the feelings associated with running, jumping, catching and throwing. Indeed, it is not simply the playing of sport that is enjoyed, but the training.

> I always feel heaps better. If I haven't trained for a couple of days, I start to feel a bit edgy and that sort of thing. I really love the peak feeling that it gives you and the feeling that you are healthy. Just being healthy

is great and I find that I get that from really pushing yourself harder. (William, aged 30, athlete)

There is now considerable scientific evidence and personal testimony that exercise makes us feel better. The first thing I found that actually helped me combat depression was running. It consistently lifted my mood and enabled me to return to life – at least for a while. I would recommend physical activity to anyone suffering from depression. When you feel like doing nothing, you need to try to do the opposite – get up and get moving. The antidepressant qualities of physical activity are a consequence of mood-enhancing chemicals such as endorphins. Physical activity also helps to burn off cortisol produced by the body when we are stressed. It is now widely understood within the psychiatric and medical communities that physical exercise is one of the most effective ways to reduce vulnerability to depression and to treat it.

THE NATURE OF EMOTION

Sport illustrates the connection between thinking (cognition), biochemistry and culture in the production of emotion. Psychiatrist Marsha Lineham describes emotions as 'full system responses'[1], by which she means that an emotion is not a single thing or event but rather involves a range of physical and mental responses. For example, fear entails a raised heartbeat, sweating, shaky limbs and increased alertness. These *physiological* features have their origins in our genetic hard wiring that developed as an evolutionary adaptation. These feelings helped us to survive by motivating us to action: the fight or flight response to danger.

However, fear is not simply a physiological response. It also involves information processing; that is, a *cognitive judgment* telling us we are in danger. For example, my brain surveys the environment and concludes that the big hairy mammoth (or 100 kilograms of muscled-up rugby forward) approaching represents a threat. Once physiological feelings are initiated, we then name them through *appraisal* mechanisms as fear, anger or love etc. Significantly, the physical dimensions of fear or anger or even love are remarkably similar, so that cognitive judgments are vital to what emotion we say we are experiencing.

Appraisals take into account the *cultural context* in which our feelings occur: if we are confronted by a tiger, we may call it fear, but if we experience similar bodily reactions to a man who has insulted us, we call it anger and if our heart is racing and our palms are sweaty in the company of someone to whom we are attracted, then we may call it love. In addition, cultural rules tell us how we may communicate our emotions; for example, whether we are allowed to express anger or not and, if we are, whether that may be through violence (for example, in boxing) or must be carefully worded (when we want to protest to the referee).

In short, thinking, physiological response and cultural naming are all constitutive of emotion; and the relationship between cognition and brain chemistry is a two-way street. Changes in our biochemistry certainly alter the way we think, as many an alcohol-induced argument or declaration of love testifies. However, neuroscience is now making it clear that changing our thoughts also changes our biochemistry. Hence, we can sometimes think ourselves into feeling happy.

Sport generates feelings of wellbeing through the biochemistry of physical activity – those endorphins again. It also entails thoughts such as 'I have done well', which lead to physiological feelings of joy and the appraisal that 'I am a worthwhile person'. It may also involve the cognition that 'I have won and I am better than you', generating pride and aggression. Thoughts of victory give rise to the physiology of jubilation, but *also* the biochemistry involved in sport gives rise to patterns of thought associated with contentment and/or triumph. Consequently, training for sportsmen needs to be physical, mental, social and emotional.

The training game

THE AUTHORITARIAN COACH

It has been suggested[2] that the power of coaches forces young men to submit to an authoritarian system of control. It is alleged that through sport men learn to regard their bodies as an instrument separated from themselves and in doing so suppress their real needs and emotions. Sport is said to train men in the ways of competition, success and violence, forging aggressive, homophobic and misogynistic cultures. One otherwise sympathetic book about men[3] has nothing good to say about sport; the author (wrongly in my view) sees only aggression and bullying.

Of course, sport can play a part in teaching men aggression and antisocial attitudes. However, this mindset can also be found in boardrooms, bedrooms, universities, nightclubs and even churches; it is not specific to sport. It is important to remember that male sporting cultures, which in any case are varied, are not simply about individual male power and violence. They are also about friendships, social networks, good habits, mentoring, self-discipline and emotional stability, as Rob argued.

ROB: THE VALUE OF SELF-DISCIPLINE

Physical, mental and emotional training is vital to sporting achievement. As a coach with responsibility for developing young rugby players, Rob told me: 'It is important to instil in them the culture that goes with rugby.' For him, this means confidence, determination, self-discipline and commitment. We might understand Rob as imposing discipline on young men in an authoritarian way. Alternatively, we might think of him as encouraging self-control and personal development.

For example, Rob encouraged players to study, develop alternative career paths, acquire personal responsibility and 'be a rounded person'. To that end, his club tries to help young players learn and grow in 'good schools and colleges'. Rob related the case of a young Indigenous player whose mother died when he was five years old and whose father is unknown. He had 'all of the cultural things that are in the way of success', including an alcohol problem. The club tried to provide for this young man by finding him a school where he would get support and develop the 'appropriate attitudes'.

Discipline is not always about the imposition of power and regulation that works-over 'docile bodies'.[4] It can also be understood as the means by which we focus attention on ourselves for the purposes of personal ethical growth and the 'care of the self'.[5] The overwhelming perspective of the sportsmen I spoke to was of the value of sporting self-control as a means of improving their lives. AFL player Rick suggested that the most important thing that he learnt at a rugby-obsessed and academically oriented grammar school was 'a good work ethic'.

The connection between sport and dedication is not unlike that found among Diggers and executives regarding effort and work (see chapter 8); namely, that it is central to their lives and identities. The upside of a devotion to 'work' is a sense of purpose and achievement. For example, Buddhism and other spiritual traditions involve shaping the character through self-discipline (see chapter 11). The downside may be a lack of healthy perspective in which other valued dimensions of life – for example, one's family – are sidelined by work. This was often the case with executives, and sometimes with sportsmen. Indeed, while I have been stressing the wellbeing of sportsmen and the value of physical activity, social connection, purpose and self-discipline, there was a darker underside for some involving fractious families, depression, drug abuse and unsatisfactory relationships.

It's a complex game: The darker side of sport

FAMILY FIGHTS: BRETT AND DAMIAN

Not all the sportsmen I talked with enjoyed secure and supportive childhood families. Brett is a 23-year-old professional basketball player. He recounted a childhood that went sour in his early teens as he clashed with his father, an authoritarian prone to bouts of bad temper. This was a tendency Brett shared with him: 'I have always had a lot of anger inside me for no apparent reason,' he said. From the age of 12, Brett began to smoke increasingly large amounts of marijuana. He started stealing and became involved in a serious incident of criminal damage, leading to an appearance in juvenile court. After a series of incidents at school, he was finally expelled. There was friction at home and things looked bleak. 'I've been depressed a lot, I guess,' he said.

But Brett was a talented basketball player who was selected for schoolboy state sides and he attracted the attention of one of Australia's prominent teams. This proved to be a turning point in his life. It was made clear to him that if he wanted to 'make it' as a professional he would have to find some self-discipline. He began to devote himself to his chosen sport and detached himself from his old friends (some of whom were now in rehab).

> I guess basketball like changed the way I lived. I realised that if I want to be a basketball player I can't do certain things. When you are playing with X there's a lot of people giving out positive information or telling you positive things and you're just around positive people. Y was telling me how much I had improved and if you do this you can really be something and that it would be silly of me not to give it a good shot. I just realised that what I was doing was a joke basically and if I played my cards right perhaps I could be good here. I told him that I was gonna do everything it takes to get me on the court and I'm glad I told him because it made me strive for something. One thing I have learnt from the numerous lectures and things I've had is to make goals and to set yourself goals, realistic goals, and to do just everything to reach them. (Brett, aged 23)

Motivated and encouraged by the club's coaching staff, Brett worked hard to hone his natural talents. Damian (aged 38), a club-based professional golfer, was less fortunate. His childhood was spent as part of a single-parent family in which his mother suffered a nervous breakdown. Though he makes a living from golf, 'I didn't have the dedication to go and do the hard yards on the golf course' in order 'to become a big player'. Instead, likeable guy though he was, Damian had alcohol, marijuana and gambling habits that threatened his health and wellbeing.

DRUGS AND ALCOHOL

Damian spoke openly about his alcohol, drug and gambling problems: 'I would drink probably every day, somewhere between, I just drink bourbon, three to six a day. If I come down to the club on a Friday night, it might be ten. I would have to consider myself bordering on the alcoholic.' In addition, Damian had been smoking marijuana every day for 20 years in tandem with the alcohol. 'It works well together,' he suggested. However, he agreed, 'there is absolutely no doubt that it interferes with golf'. Further, according to Damian, 'gambling is definitely a culture in golf, all the way from Tiger Woods down to the juniors. You have got to have a bet, you can't play for nothing.' Damian was now working to resolve his debt problem, since 'in my yesteryear I used to gamble a lot'.

Another professional basketball player, Louis (aged 33), had avoided drinking and smoking marijuana when he was at school 'out of respect for my high school coach'. But when he went to college 'the whole basketball team got together and we started drinking and man that was a good night and I couldn't wait to do it again'. Louis developed a drinking habit. He claimed never to drink at least 24 hours before a game. Nonetheless, post-match drinking was a frequent occurrence that continued until the bar closed in the early hours of the morning. His wife thought he drank too much and stayed out too late.

The relationship game

Though sport has a strong social dimension, a powerful commitment to it may also restrict intimate relationships. As Rob noted, male sporting comradeship did not often extend into the realms of personal support in the face of thorny emotions. 'I've worked with many men and getting males to open up is really difficult,' he observed. Indeed, where sportsmen did conform to the conventional view was in their attitude towards women. Only a few had developed long-term relationships with women who were often, though not always, peripheral to their lives.

MITCH AND JEFF: IT'S A BATTLE

The commitment required to 'achieve' at high levels in sport can put relationships with partners, wives and girlfriends under stress (a pattern similar to corporate executives – see chapter 8). Mitch (aged 35) suggested that, in order to play professional cricket, 'you need a very supportive partner, who in turn has to create a life for themselves. It's not easy'. Professional sportsmen are away from home a considerable amount of time. In Mitch's case, there was also a good deal of uncertainty about his career and with it the family's finances. Nevertheless, he had remained married for nine years and he and his wife had three children. 'I think it's been an absolute battle. It's been an up-and-down marriage, but we have been through a lot together and that's the bond we have,' he said.

Similarly, Jeff maintained that 'nothing in terms of two people living together is bloody successful' and described his marriage as 'a constant battle'. He linked a philosophy of sport to his life and relationships:

> It's not easy and it's about overcoming difficulties and if you can do that you'll succeed and that's the same thing for life as well. Life is not easy, if you are willing to overcome difficulties you'll be all right, so that means every time something is difficult you have to have the mentality to overcome it and you'll be fine. The moment that you think things should work for you, or they don't work for you and you think you should give up, you're doomed. (Jeff, aged 44)

Some young men found that their commitment to sport was incompatible with long-term relationships. None of basketball coach Martin's girlfriends had remained with him for more than a few months because of his dedication to sport. Likewise, Alex said that he 'never had any trouble getting girlfriends', but found that he was always the one who ended the relationships. Since this was upsetting, he had decided to put partnerships aside until he was older. Certainly, the 'positive' profile of sport presented by these men was somewhat undermined by their attitudes to women and relationships. But then the same could be said of many young men, including highly educated university students.

LOUIS: YOU DON'T OWN ME

Pro-basketball player Louis offered a justification for why marriage and relationships can't work because they imply 'ownership' of others: 'The way we have got them set up, they can't work, they're just too limited. Okay, so now we go out together and now you think you own me and I'm yours and I gotta ring you, and if I go two days without ringing you, it's "How come you didn't ring me?".' He favoured relationships that were 'open: no obligations, no rules' (Louis, aged 33).

Louis may have a point about possessiveness as a destructive force in relationships. The trouble is, Louis was married with children and was justifying his willingness to have sex with other women. He argued that since this was also an option for his wife (claiming this would not upset him), and because he planned to remain with her, then 'I don't call that cheating'. Of course, Louis had not told his wife about his extramarital sexual activity and she had not taken up her option to do likewise! Louis's childhood had not, however, offered him a model for a loving partnership (see chapter 4), quite the reverse: 'One thing my father told me that I'll never forget is don't let a woman make you afraid to be a man.'

CRAIG: ONE OF THE GOOD GUYS

Craig told me that girlfriends 'don't always understand everything it takes to be a professional footballer'. In particular, he felt that the team bonding facets of the game, from which women are excluded, could be upsetting to them. In his view, players needed to be honest with their partners about the demands of professional sport and if necessary 'stand up' for what they have to do. Partners, he said, should be supportive of players and help them in their career. He didn't mention the reverse possibility.

According to Craig, many footballers choose to be single rather than enter a steady relationship because of the demands of the game, and 'because there are more girls on hand, if you know what I mean'. Indeed, rugby league in Australia has struggled with a series of incidents (including sexual violence), leading commentators to label the sport as intrinsically misogynistic. However, it might equally be said that the attitudes of footballers are no different from those of other young men, but that their celebrity status has given them more sexual 'opportunities'. For his part, Craig told me that football had never been a problem for him and his partner. As I left his house, he commented to his girlfriend that we had discussed football and relationships. She laughed and said: 'He is one of the good guys, you know.'

The sports screen

In this chapter, I have stressed the uplifting side of male sport. I attributed the above-average levels of emotional wellbeing experienced by these sportsmen to constructive patterns of thought, sustained social connections, a sense of purpose, physical health and self-discipline. The positive psychology of happiness[6] also evaluates these features as vital to our contentment (see chapter 10). Psychology suggests that the most important factor in determining happiness is our social connection with others. In a parallel fashion, Buddhism can also be understood as a set of self-disciplined trainings that improve the quality of life (see chapter 11). Perhaps we could even talk about the spirituality of sport.

Yet, the popular image of sportsmen behaving badly under the influence of alcohol is not entirely without foundation. Nor is the sense that professional sport is a male-dominated world that is hostile to women groundless. Further, some sportsmen get depressed and others are unable to deal with their anger. It is important to say, however, that these troubles were less pronounced among the sportsmen I spoke with than among other groups of men. I suspect that sport has become the screen onto which we project our fears and anxieties about men and emotion in our culture. We might be better served by worrying less about sport and asking ourselves why it is we are talking so much about men and their emotions at all right now. This is the theme of our next chapter.

Why we are talking about men now

At the age of 15, Trevor left home to live on the streets of 'The Cross', a slice of Sydney that houses the sex industry, drug users and organised crime. He fell into 'the seedy side of life', working as a doorman at sex clubs where his social circle comprised sex workers, strippers, bouncers and bikers. At 17, he 'hooked up with Hells Angels and really got involved in the club. We did pills, dope, a bit of coke, mostly acid and a lot of drinking; yeah, a lot of violence. We were involved in a lot of violence'.

Social alarm about the key features of Trevor's story – drugs, alcohol, violence, macho men's clubs and the feral side of sex – is one of the reasons why Western culture is currently engaged in a conversation about men. There is growing concern about men's aggressive and violent relationships with others; their predilection for addiction to drugs, alcohol and sex; an apparent increase in mental health difficulties that looks like an epidemic of depression, and a sense that men have become unsure about their place in the world. In short, there is a feeling that men in Western cultures are caught up in an emotional crisis.

There is more to be learnt from Trevor's story, however, than the simple facts of sex, drugs and bikers. There is, for example, the abiding significance of social connection and of family:

> The one thing I found with the club is the comradeship. You feel like you belong. It's the only place where I've really learnt what family means. People may think it's strange because they don't see the family values; they don't see any family association at all, but a Hells Angel will put his family first and foremost. And they are loyal to one another. They will never do wrong by one another. (Trevor, aged 47)

Trevor stumbled upon a warmth of human relationships with the family of Hells Angels that he had not found in his own childhood. He explained that he 'had a very emotional and to some extent physically abusive childhood'. He was continually told that he would never amount to anything, that he was 'no good, useless and lazy'. He was never once told that he was loved nor cuddled or kissed. His parents were both alcoholics and he repeatedly witnessed them argue violently: 'They used to attack each other with carving knives, broken beer bottles, anything they could get their hands on. I've got scars on me from where I've been belted, but they are only superficial; nothing like the scars that I've got emotionally.'

In due course, Trevor distanced himself from the Hells Angels to live a more conventional life of marriage and children. But while it was possible to leave his biker family behind, the same was not true of his childhood. Sadly, but predictably, Trevor's family of origin followed him into his adult relationships, where he reproduced the violence and alcohol abuse enacted by his parents. Inevitably, divorce and separation from his children ensued. Increasingly, cultural awareness of the emotional damage that parents can inflict on their children, along with the historically high divorce rate and the prevalence of fatherless children, underpins our anxiety about the family and fuels apprehension towards men. Social concern about absent fathers, male violence and drug abuse are themes of both the media and contemporary writing about men, as we shall see below.

TALKING PSYCHOLOGY

Trevor continued to embody the reasons for our cultural disquiet: he married again and began 'sabotaging our relationship by drinking heavily'. However, Trevor was more fortunate on this occasion; his new wife understood the root causes of his behaviour and encouraged him to attend counselling.

> I went and saw a psychologist for about four or five months and got to the stage where I could talk about my childhood. I was brought up in such a way that I couldn't talk. If I had something wrong inside, if something was bothering me, I couldn't talk about it and these nightmares were going on, oh, I dunno, over ten years, I suppose. They had been going on and I hadn't told anybody. (Trevor, aged 47)

Trevor found psychotherapy useful to him in building up his self-esteem and developing communication skills. He described how he and his wife were now able to sit down and talk with each other for hours on end. 'It's everything I've ever looked for in a relationship,' he said.

Now, the widespread diffusion of psychological ideas throughout our culture, courtesy of self-help literature and television shows like *Oprah*, is a double-edged sword. On the one hand, our increased awareness of psychological dynamics is valuable for men like Trevor and me. On the other hand, it fuels a widespread anxiety that our emotional lives are permanently in difficulty and require attention. Either way, our increased use of a psychological vocabulary is a significant driver in the contemporary conversation about men.

In particular, it has become an axiom that men are unable to express their emotions, and that this is detrimental to their relationships. It is now widely accepted that men 'suppress' their emotions. Trevor does seem to agree. Nonetheless, we may note that he *had* been expressing his prickly emotions – through alcohol and violence. It is not that he wasn't expressing emotion, but that he was not doing so in a socially approved or personally productive way. We feel (and I agree) that talking about challenging emotions is more valuable than acting them out in destructive ways. It was learning to talk about emotion in a particular way that Trevor found beneficial. The key issue, then, is not whether men can express emotion, but how they do so.

It is significant that Trevor's wife encouraged him to see a therapist, and that the measure of his achievement was his ability to communicate with her. In part, it is women's rising expectations of greater intimacy and their disappointments that lie behind our social unease towards men. During the past 50 years, women have campaigned for, and to some degree achieved, greater levels of social and economic equality. They now understandably want a commensurate level of emotional democracy within their relationships. And they are saying so.

As it happens, Trevor's marriage was somewhat unconventional since his wife was bisexual and had been politically active within the lesbian community. He feared he might lose her to another woman: 'But when I talked about it to her, it was okay and we worked it out.' Increasingly, the complexity of contemporary life involves negotiating the terms of our relationships, and this requires us to learn the vocabulary and skills to do so.

The tribulations of depression, alcoholism and violence that men experience do not suggest a lack of emotion or its suppression per se, but rather excess. Indeed, it has been suggested that men possess more reactive biologically based emotional systems than do women.[1] In any case, men do not always communicate their emotions in the most skilful way. Attention should be paid then to men's emotional vocabulary and its consequences, particularly given the growing evidence of their emotional and psychological suffering.

SYMPTOMS OF DISTRESS

In the United States, some 48 per cent of men are implicated in depression, suicide, alcoholism, drug abuse, violence and crime at some point in their lives.[2] In Australia, a government health survey (*Sun Herald*, 29 August 1999) found that men are more likely than women to be obese, to have an accident (five times higher) and be diagnosed as HIV-positive (ten times higher). Men are also more likely than women to be diagnosed as having 'mental disorders' as a child (for example, attention deficit disorder), engage in high-risk behaviour (for example, dangerous levels of drinking or drug taking) and be a victim of suicide (six times higher, with 80 per cent of suicide victims being male and death rates highest among men aged 20–24 or 80 and above).

According to writer and activist Steve Biddulph[3], there are few happy men. For him, the central problems of men's lives are loneliness, compulsive competition and lifelong emotional timidity. These characteristics are rooted, he suggests, in the adoption of impossible images of masculinity that men try, but fail, to live up to. British psychiatrist Anthony Clare[4] points out that throughout North America, Europe and Australia male suicides outnumber those committed by women by between three and four to one. For every six elderly women that kill themselves, 40 elderly men will take their own lives, while the number of young male suicides is at epidemic proportions. This supports Warren Farrell's[5] depiction of men as the 'disposable gender' who are slaughtered in wars, commit suicide more often than women and are the victims of violence, overwork and mental illness.

Clare also suggests that men are increasingly subject to a variety of health problems that have received less public attention than they warrant, including cancer, anxiety, depression, circulatory problems and HIV-related disorders. Among the many factors that account for this is the tendency for men to be more *isolated* psychologically and socially than women (see chapter 9).

MALE VIOLENCE

The problem of violence is largely a problem of men. Clare reports that a man is over 20 times more likely to kill another man than a woman is to kill a woman and a man is more likely to kill a woman than a woman is to kill a man. In England and Wales in 1989, there were seven times more indictable offences recorded against men than against women. Across the Western world, men commit over 90 per cent of convicted acts of violence and comprise over 90 per cent of the inmates of jails.

> I started drinking, smoking and hanging around the boys in Redfern [a suburb of Sydney with a significant Indigenous population] and that's where I felt comfortable, 'cause I'm Koori [Indigenous Australian] as well and they taught me how to car thieve and do all sorts of crime, smash

and grabs, armed robbery ... I hung around the boys in Redfern and then I got locked up for car stealing. I was right in there because 70 per cent were Kooris and they all look after each other, make sure you are comfortable and have got drugs, they'll fix you up. When I got out of Long Bay [prison], when I felt like taking my life, I got all better, 'cause the boys gave me strength. (Toby, aged 31)

Signs of male distress fuel the contemporary identification of men as a social problem, for themselves and for others. Every culture involves 'discourses' or patterned ways of speaking and thinking about men that contain expectations of male behaviour. This is what is meant by the idea of 'masculinity' – the ways we represent men and what we expect of them. Discourses of masculinity shape how men understand themselves and are understood by others. However, many of the long-standing ways through which men have recognised themselves may no longer be serving us well.

MASCULINITY AS A PROBLEM

A good deal of literature now describes 'masculinity' as a problem for men[6], a sentiment echoed by popular magazines and television. The argument goes like this. Men work too hard these days, becoming stressed and ill in the process. We fail to look after our health because we have learnt to see ourselves as invulnerable. Having been taught that our duty is to work hard for our families, we overlook our own wellbeing. Men, we are told, become psychologically committed to achievement in order to please their imaginary fathers and prop up their fragile sense of self-worth.

In preparation for the pursuit of success, it is said, men have been told that it is 'a dog-eat-dog world out there' and that they must use all means available to reach the top. Personal competitive power is valued over co-operation. Consequently, men lack intimate male friends because they have been taught to be competitive with each other. In addition, it is claimed that men have not developed the proactive skills to build social networks because they have learnt that independence and self-reliance are accorded greater value. The outcome is that men become socially isolated and discontented.

Our culture has largely accepted the view that men value action over reflection and that they are more inclined to 'do' than 'be', to act rather than to talk. This tendency is linked to men's training in 'rationality' and stoicism ('be a man'), a corollary of which is the claimed unwillingness or inability of men to talk about their emotions. Certainly, men are not always able to talk productively about emotions like love, grief and fear because they have not learnt the appropriate vocabulary. This can make men's intimate relationships with women thornier, especially given our cultural history of seeing women as objects of desire rather than as fully human. However, the most damaging aspect of masculinity today, or so psychology tells us, are the feelings of inadequacy we develop about ourselves because we are unable to live up to our own ideals. It is this feeling of defectiveness that fuels alcohol and drug abuse.

There is much to be said for these arguments in relation to many, though not all, men. In the rest of this book, we will witness many examples of men thinking and behaving in these ways. For example, we will hear about executives who work long hours and neglect their families. We will meet young homeless boys and hardworking family men who are socially isolated, depressed and who turn to the temporary haven of drugs and alcohol. We will listen to old men and young talking about their long histories of troubled relationships with women in which they repeat the same mistakes.

Nevertheless, we will also encounter men rejecting these cultural rules and seeking alternative ways to live. We will hear about men who are developing more open and democratic relationships with women. We will meet men who have turned their back on overwork to pursue other interests and talk with men who have beaten addiction to find a new, more contented, path in life. What all these men have in common is that, successfully or traumatically, they are learning that deeply held ideas about what it is to be a man are inadequate for living contentedly in the modern world. Ways of being long understood by men to be natural and acceptable are now thought of as 'a problem' because the social context in which we act as men has changed.

Social change and modern men

The place that men hold in the world is increasingly uncertain. Until recently, we have taken our position in the social order as men for granted. We did not need to ask ourselves what it meant to be a man or how men should behave. This is not to say that we did not ask questions about 'the meaning of life'. Rather, it is to suggest that these questions and their answers were not posed in terms of being a man. The current period is the first in which we are being forced to ask about what it actually means to live as a man. James, a psychotherapist by profession, told me about his experience of talking with men:

> There is so much uncertainty out there amongst men. About how to behave with women, you know. What should you do? Is opening the door for a woman polite or are you gonna get it shut in your face? Do you work your guts out for the family or stay at home with the kids? And even if you want to, can you afford to? Do you even know what to do? And losing your job can be devastating. I have seen that a few times. When that happens, many men just aren't sure who they are or what they are worth anymore. (James, aged 48)

We are living through a period when old and trusted maps of meaning are giving way to the uncertainties of a new order. Men now have to confront questions about masculinity because the ground of prior certainty is being cut away from them by a series of social and cultural changes. These multidimensional interlinked changes concern the economy, technology, politics, culture and identities. Of particular significance here are the changes associated with work, family and the conduct of relationships.

CHANGE AT WORK

Upheavals in the global economy over the last 30 years have brought many changes to the world of work. Western economies have experienced a shift from manufacturing towards service industries and the information economy. Consequently, we are witnessing a decline in the manual working class, a rise in service and white-collar work, and an increase in part-time labour. Simultaneously, we have seen the creation of a new 'underclass' of the unemployed and unemployable.

Changes in the economy have affected men in varied ways. The manual working class and 'underclass' have been particularly badly hit by the loss of skills, income and self-worth. To some degree, the 'crisis of masculinity' is a calamity of the working-class man who had found his social value and self-worth through being *useful* at work and to his family, and now finds himself without a job and without a purpose. The man who expected to be in control and who made things happen became superfluous. In her survey of American men, feminist author Susan Faludi[7] documents a series of 'men in trouble', from shipyard workers who have lost both their income and their craftsmanship, pride and solidarity to corporate executives watching their consumer dream of the house, the pool, the car and the cosy family threatened by economic downturn.

At the same time, our 21st-century consumer culture obliges those of us in work to acquire more and more income to spend on the things we want. We live in a world of advertising whose central message is buy, buy and buy some more because we are inadequate just as we are. We feel we must have this car, this house and this item of clothing in order to be of worth. Shopping is an emotional experience that temporarily makes us feel good, but whose 'high' is inevitably short-lived. Then we need to spend again and so we need to earn yet more. Across the Western world, we are working longer and longer hours. For example, new working practices, including rising levels of surveillance, have increased the workload for middle-class white-collar workers who regularly work 50-, 60- or even 70-hour weeks.

> I must spend the greater part of my life in the office these days. You know, I work 12 and 14-hour days on a regular basis during the week and at least part of the weekend. I try to put aside family time on Sundays, but there is always something to be done. That's the nature of the job and you know it's long hours but I also get a buzz from it or I wouldn't do it. Though sometimes I wonder about whether it's worth it. But that's just a bad day and it passes (Frank, aged 43).

When men work such long hours, it is difficult for them to fully participate in their family life even when they want to, as many increasingly do. And our intensified working hours are not providing us with the sense of purpose and meaning that we need. According to Faludi, the Second World War proved to be the 'last gasp' of the useful and dutiful male as the ideal of manhood. In particular, the culture of celebrity, image, entertainment and marketing, underpinned by consumerism, signalled the end of 'usefulness' as the measure of men. Masculinity has become a matter of personal display rather than the demonstration of 'internal' qualities of moral strength, confidence and purpose. Consequently, 'the boy who had been told he was going to be the master of the universe and all that was in it found himself master of nothing'.[8]

In the absence of an alternative vision of manhood that could provide a new sense of meaning and purpose, men have lost their way. For example, Faludi describes Christian men who try to reassert their symbolic status as head of the family even as their wives pack and leave. Like her, I found young men who seek wealth and purpose in consumer culture and, failing to find either, turn instead to crime; and I met executives who, despite their social status and income, were depressed and drank to excess. Nevertheless, I also talked to older men whose working career had given them a sense of meaning, and to men who were finding a new purpose beyond the confines of work.

THE CHANGING FAMILY

Today we are experiencing tensions between love, family and personal freedom that are restructuring the family. We seek love, but if our family doesn't work out as we hoped, we are prepared to break it apart to renew the quest. In searching for a right way to live, we put our individual desires above those of other people. We try out cohabitation, divorce or living on our own. We struggle to coordinate family and career, love and marriage, friendships and community.

These changes are marked by historically high divorce figures, the sharp rise in informal or de facto marriages and the increasing number of people who live alone. The Australian Bureau of Statistics reports

(Media Release 3310.0, 22 August 2002) that fewer people are choosing to marry and more couples are choosing to cohabit. The median age at marriage is increasing and the number of divorces is increasing. There is mounting evidence that marriage is good for men's health, yet by 2010 one in three men will be living alone.[9] More and more children live in families without fathers.

> I didn't understand why my dad wasn't there and why my mum had to go to work; basically I just didn't understand. I missed out on a hell of a lot, you know, going to the footy with my dad, things like that and just mucking around. My dad used to ride motorbikes and things like that and he used to always come home with the skin off him. I do the same with pushbikes; it's fun. (Brian, aged 22)

There are writers and politicians who claim that the absence of fathers in children's lives accounts for poverty, rising juvenile crime, eating disorders, suicide, depression, drug abuse and other social problems. They maintain that children who grow up with one parent are more likely to become teen mothers, to drop out of school and become unemployed. However, this point of view is controversial. It is just as likely that parental conflict and poverty (which often accompanies single parenthood) accounts for these difficulties rather than changes in family form per se.

It is true that the quality of childhood relationships is the cornerstone of our later emotional health. That is the overwhelming implication of this book. However, my investigations lead me to concur with family researcher Judith Stacey[10], who suggests that children do not need any specific kind of family life so much as they need loving, nurturing, caring adults; and this can occur in a variety of forms. I certainly found that men from chaotic and unhappy families were more likely to be depressed alcoholics in later life. Sometimes these were fatherless families, but equally often they were not. I also encountered men from single-parent families who were happy and emotionally stable.

My own family remained intact, but this did not prevent me experiencing depression and a difficult relationship with my father, whose own childhood was supervised by both parents. The conventional two-parent family has a long history of violence, the subordination of women and child abuse laying the foundations of 'mental illness'. There is no doubt that the family is undergoing change and that this is the cause of some disorientation. However, the solutions do not lie in a mythical return to the 'family values' of the 1950s, but rather in finding new ways to live together and raise children.

Change is always difficult to live with, but a sense of bewilderment about contemporary family life is particularly strong among men because women are driving the revolution in relationships. Men must adapt, sometimes with difficulty, to women's desire for greater equality and openness in relationships.

CHANGING RELATIONSHIPS

Marriage and the family have long been based on inequality between men and women. The 'traditional' 1950s allocation of family responsibilities made men the breadwinners and women the homemakers. Women still do not enjoy full social and political equality with men. However, since the mid-1960s there have been significant changes in the relationship between men and women. Women have made notable gains in the economy, where they make up a larger percentage of the workforce and are paid better than they once were. Women are more visible in the world of business and politics (though still in a significant minority) as well as in the cultural sphere as writers, artists and actors.

There have also been changes in sexual attitudes and behaviour by which women have more autonomy and command greater respect. Reform of divorce laws has allowed women to escape oppressive relationships more easily, and women initiate the vast majority of divorces. Gender inequality and gender injustice are still evident. Nevertheless, many of the central tenets of feminism have been absorbed into our culture. Of particular significance is a transformation in the way we now expect relationships between men and women to be conducted.

Relationships can no longer rely on the law or the Church or the extended family or force or lack of choice to hold them together. Divorce is relatively easy to obtain, religion has lost its moral sway over the majority of Western populations, and kinship networks are flung far and wide. Although domestic violence remains entrenched, we at least publicly condemn it, while greater economic independence allows more women to flee from aggressive husbands. Increasingly, then, we must *justify* the continuation of relationships rather than simply accept the continuation of family arrangements that make us unhappy.

It is a growing challenge to say with any clear authority how marriage, parenthood, sexuality or love must be organised or what they mean. There is no longer a pre-eminent model of how relationships should work that we are obliged to follow. Rather, relationships are increasingly matters of individual negotiation. They have to be worked out, discussed and justified in all their particularistic details. Personal autonomy, trust, reciprocity and equality are increasingly necessary characteristics of relationships, which must acknowledge in theory, if not always in practice, the requirement for greater democracy.[11]

The modern family has conventionally required men to be independent and outward-looking. This comes at the price of a masked emotional dependence on women and weaker skills of emotional communication. The long-standing predominance of men in the economic domain has left the 'emotion work' of family intimacy to women. Consequently, many men lack skills of emotion management adequate to the new times in which we are experimenting with relationships that are more democratic.

> I married. I didn't have very good social skills, naturally enough, being rejected a lot as a child. I was very very fearful of being rejected. So, almost I ended up marrying the first girl I went out with, at the age of 21. She was 18 and I was 21 and we got married and I was highly neurotic, very fearful, very jealous, very insecure and violent. I would lose my temper and strike her maybe four or five times a year. I never put her in hospital or never bruised her. There was a certain amount of control there but I was abusive and guilt was not part of my self-image. (Mike, aged 57)

As women pioneer radical changes in our private lives that challenge the taken-for-granted cultural practices of male control, so men are wondering about how they should conduct relationships. Some men struggle to make sense of relationships with women or to talk to their partners in the most productive way and thus hinder the development of emotionally democratic relationships. However, so far as this is the case, we need to understand it not simply as the operation of male power in defence of the status quo, but also as a moment of confusion and emotional pain. We don't just 'understand' what is expected of us as a man through our self-conscious talk, but more importantly we *feel* an emotional connection with descriptions of 'how to be a man' (though we may also contest them). As the old stories of manhood become discredited, we should take this as an opportunity to profitably make ourselves anew, but for many there is a significant sense of loss.

Masculinity: Attachment and loss

As infants, we are born into a dangerous and uncertain world in which we feel vulnerable and at risk. We need our parents to care for us and so we form bonds of attachment that, when they work well, enable us to venture securely into the world. However, where such attachments are insecure or under threat, we feel anxious, afraid and angry. As we grow older and more independent, we transfer some of our need for attachment and security onto other people (most notably women as love objects for heterosexual men).

There is an analogous process at work when we adopt stories about the world in order to explain it. Believing in the solidity of our cultural maps of meaning and emotionally identifying with them makes us feel safe. Knowing how to go on in the world as a man makes us feel secure, even if those stories no longer generate desirable consequences. For example, many men feel safe in the knowledge that they are hardworking men even when their families complain about their absence or they are suffering from stress-related illnesses. Conversely, when we are faced with the loss of the old stories and are unable to find any comforting new stories to take their place, we tend to suffer.

HOLDING ON AND LETTING GO

There are ways of being a man that have always posed problems for us. For example, we have continually suffered and died in war through our attachment to duty, stoical toughness and invulnerability. Yet, these qualities were not seen as damaging to men as men; that is, as an issue of masculinity. What makes the contemporary condition unique is that long-standing ways of living as a man are being undermined by the wider cultural changes discussed above. A sense of loss and disorientation arises as men recognise the need to change – or are forced to do so – but have not yet forged new secure ways to be.

Some men experience diminished self-worth and insecurity as their place in the economy and authority as 'head of the family' is undermined. Other men undergo confusion and loss as their emotional dependence on women is questioned. Carrying out their own 'emotion work' in relationships and forging emotional bonds with children and friends can be a challenge. More subtly, women now expect greater emotional literacy and more skilful management of relationships from men than previously. In that context, continued attachment to a masculinity that asserts male power at the expense of women blocks dialogue and leads to emotional suffering. If men hang on to the old stories, their relationships will flounder; but if they seek to change themselves, they face a period of insecurity. It takes courage to transform oneself.

Conflicting expectations of behaviour can lead men to feel insecure and confused. For example, men are now expected to play a greater role in the upbringing of children and to value being a father more strongly. Yet, increasingly large numbers of men are separated from their children by divorce and the termination of relationships. Men are also expected to work longer and longer hours, which they do in search of success, a required male behaviour. However, long hours at work are not compatible with their equally anticipated engagement with childcare.

Change is often a difficult and painful process. Nevertheless, the redesigning of 'what it is to be a man' can be grasped in positive and beneficial ways. We are currently presented with the opportunity to constructively reshape masculinity: to value others more, to improve our relationships with women and children, to downgrade the place of paid work and owning objects. We have the opportunity to develop new ways of being a man, or rather new ways to be human, which bring respect, esteem and contentment. To succeed, we need to understand how men speak about emotions – the core theme of this book. To do that, we must first examine the place of emotion talk in our lives.

Experience and emotion talk

There is a dimension of emotion that we can't quite grasp with words. Emotions appear to just happen to us; we are often not self-consciously aware of the cognitive and physiological processes involved. Even when we are aware of our 'experiences', our attention is brought to bear on the component parts of an emotion rather than 'an emotion'. That is, we experience physiological feelings (e.g. a racing heart and sweaty palms) along with thought patterns such as: 'You are a threat to me'. We do not experience 'fear' or 'anger' as distinct entities, because no such entities exist. Rather, these concepts are labels that we apply as shorthand ways of grasping our experiences.

Emotions motivate us to action. They are a mode of being or a form of 'embodied consciousness' that we exist through, but which may nevertheless be outside of our conscious attention. Nonetheless, we give meaning to our awareness of emotion through language, which 'points to' aspects of our direct embodied experience. We can understand emotions as bodily sensations and actions that are made meaningful through poetic metaphors.

For example, when we speak about emotion we often deploy metaphors of heat and cold, pressure and release, flow and stasis, and so on. We talk about someone as being 'hot-tempered' or describe an emotionally inexpressive person as being a 'cold fish'. We may say that we 'blew our top' or that we are 'filled' with love. We also use spatial metaphors, often related to the body. Thus we feel 'up' or 'down', we are hurt 'inside' or we want to get our anger 'out'. Jake, who we met in chapter 1, described the need to metaphorically 'get it out' through talking about his feelings:

> It's good to get it out because if I keep it inside it boils up and then once it boils up anything can trigger it and once it triggers I go into a suicidal mood where I just start hitting things and punching myself in the face, so it's best that I get it out anyway. (Jake, aged 23)

Culture provides us with the language we use to think about emotion and to 'let it out'. Human emotions are culturally constructed to the degree that languages name and give meaning to the experiences we call 'emotions'; and thus give rise to particular patterns of thinking. In that sense, emotions are constituted by the way we talk about them. They are part of a shared repertoire of explanations and maps of meaning rather than being generated from within individuals.

JAKE'S EMOTIONS ARE CULTURAL

Jake suffered from despair brought about by the way he thinks of himself as hopeless. It is likely that he is constantly ruminating on the difficulties in his life and that he has a harshly self-critical internal voice. These unfavourable self-judgments may even represent 'conclusions' (as neurological pathways) that he came to during his pre-verbal childhood. However, they are now expressed through a language that involves 'taking inside' cultural values manifested as the 'inner parent'. Indeed, he described: 'a war going on inside myself' between creative and destructive voices.

Subsequently, Jake learnt through the language of psychology to describe his complex amalgam of thoughts and feelings as depression. This cultural naming makes Jake's emotions available to management and treatment. It forges a swirling array of thoughts and feelings into a 'thing'. Treatment for Jake's named 'condition' involves training him how to express his feelings in culturally acceptable ways. In particular, he was urged not to use drugs or violence as a way to manage his emotions. To this end, he was introduced to writing and drama as ways to develop wisdom about his emotions (from which he also gained enjoyment and self-confidence).

> I've been writing poetry and I've been looking back over periods, looking at what happened here and there. I came first in a competition here in poetry and I was in hospital at the time too. It felt like people could understand what my problems are about. It was about my feelings of everyday life. So I explained my feelings and it came out number one. Then I started helping with *Big Heart*, going around doing drama in schools. (Jake, aged 23)

Our ways of speaking about emotion are integrated into the stories of our lives through a double movement. Emotion talk involves both an attempt to grasp the direct experience of the moment using metaphors and an integration of that moment into a narrative of the past and future. Emotion is given meaning in the context of our life stories and itself gives our life stories meaning.

EMOTION AND IDENTITY STORIES

We generally think that our emotional responses form a significant part of who we are. Stories about emotion are thus an important feature of our identities. Identity is not a fixed eternal essence of a person. Identity is not a thing at all. Rather, identity is simply a meaningful description we give to ourselves. Just like Jake above, and Peter below, we construct our identity through telling the stories of our lives through, for example, tales of romantic love.

> I never thought much of myself as an emotional kind of man. I thought of myself as a businessman. Of course, I had feelings, but the centre of my life was work and feelings about work. I guess I knew I was a bit lonely too and I had half an eye out for the possibility of meeting someone and I sort of felt I was a bit odd as well, to be honest, because I wasn't married but I tried to keep that at arm's length. Now I think of myself as a married man and a family man and work is still important, but it's kind of shifted a bit more to the edge. (Peter, aged 45)

As Peter tells a story about his emotional life, so he constructs and performs his identity. Now, our culture gives us quite particular ways of talking about 'men and emotion' to draw on when we speak. These 'scripts' or 'discourses' are made up of statements that tell us 'how to be a man'. In this way, culture gives us rules that prescribe what we can say or think about men. For example, it is not conventionally allowed to positively evaluate a man as 'emotional'. An emotional man is commonly regarded as weak and/or feminine.

Of course, our ideas about men and emotion are not static but change over time. During the 1950s, men were conventionally described as unemotional and/or required to keep their emotions 'inside'. 'Boys don't cry' was the watchword. However, contemporary culture is increasingly demanding that men should talk about their emotions. In particular, men are being asked to acquire a language of love and intimacy on the one hand and the means to control anger and violence on the other.

Institutional practices of masculinity are also culturally specific. In professional sport, it is entirely acceptable to express powerful emotions at an intense moment of triumph or defeat. One may shed a tear at the end of a cup final. However, in more everyday contexts – for example, crying at the movies – such behaviour is frowned upon and subject to group discipline. The 'overly emotional' man is likely to be ostracised by other sportsmen. Similarly, there is little room for open talk about depression in the boardrooms of corporate business. To do so is to risk being perceived as not being up to the job.

Public reactions to male tears have, of course, changed as evolving attitudes to postwar politicians illustrate. Britain's wartime Prime Minister Winston Churchill is known to have suffered from debilitating bouts of depression. Yet, Churchill never cried in public and it is inconceivable that his political career could have survived had he done so. In 1972, US Senator Ed Muskie's public tears derailed his campaign for the Democratic Party presidential nomination. So damaging was his display of emotion that he attributed the dampness of his cheeks to snowflakes. However, by the 1980s Bob Hawke, the long-serving Australian Prime Minister, was able to cry in public on a number of occasions without damaging his career, despite it being founded on being 'one of the boys'. By the end of the 20th century, Bill Clinton had turned strategic weeping into a political art form.

It would seem, then, that it is now more acceptable for men to cry in public. Nonetheless, the reasons attributed to men's tears play a significant part in their cultural reception. When Hawke cried tears of sadness for his drug-addicted daughter, there was public sympathy. But when the tears seemed to flow too often and for less compelling reasons, there were questions about the role alcohol played in his life. In other words, a form of cultural discipline still governs the expression of emotion.

How our culture teaches us to think about men is not one-dimensional; there are competing ways of speaking about masculinity, so that each particular man negotiates between different scripts or discourses. We are simultaneously both the product of our culture and unique individuals, just as all snowflakes are made of H_2O but each is distinctive. All men experience emotions and can in varying ways also speak about emotions. But men are not all the same and the precise way of speaking that each of us deploys has singular consequences. That is why we need to explore the emotion talk of particular men, the situations that invoke emotions for them and the male behaviours that their languages of emotion seek to explain.

MAN TROUBLE

At the dawn of the 21st century, the place and status of men in Western culture is coming under scrutiny. In particular, men are facing new challenges associated with changes in the nature of work and the conduct of relationships. In this context, a number of men are experiencing difficulties of a psychological and emotional character that manifest themselves through depression and drug or alcohol abuse. Some of these difficulties stem from the power of long-standing facets of 'being a man', while others flow from changes that have undermined modern 'masculinity'. In any case, emotion must be at the core of any investigation into the lives of contemporary men because it is central to their experience of social and personal transformation. Now it is the difficulties that men have with their emotions and subsequent self-destructive behaviour that has caught the headlines. Young homeless drug users are a group of men with a high media profile who stand out as signs of our troubled times. It is to my conversations with these men that we now turn.

Your mum and dad

Can Marcus ever recover?

Trouble called on Marcus at a young age. He had his first joint at the age of 13 and, after increasing conflict with his teachers, he was expelled from school. His father tried, and failed, to beat him into submission. At 17, Marcus ran away from his violent family life for an equally tough one on the city streets. He was homeless and a heroin addict. To survive, he and his girlfriend resorted to crime and prostitution.

> Ever since then, me and [Jane] done it hard, and I mean hard. We have lived on the street. We lived on the street for two whole years. She had to degrade herself; she had to work as a prostitute while being with me. I've had to degrade myself. Being on drugs, being on hammer [heroin] you'll do anything and that's the hard thing. I've done it a few times, I pulled in more money than her, a guy does. For an hour it was two hundred bucks and I was just looking after my habit, you know. Now I cry my eyes out. To make myself feel better, I have to shove a needle in my arm and degrade myself. We've both done it and cried for days. You

> get to the point where you'd even rob some old lady for that too. Thank God it never came to that. (Marcus, aged 20)

I met Marcus at the drop-in centre for 'at risk' young men and women, where he recounted his poignant and distressing tale. It became clear that the emotional anguish of family disturbance formed the backdrop to his troubled and chaotic life. Marcus's father was a harsh disciplinarian, prone to excessive drinking and violence, who tried to control his wife and sons through beatings. Both his parents were heavy drinkers.

> He was a drinker and me mum was too and it was a very violent relationship between them and my mum left with all of us kids. The last thing I remember is a big big big fight and my mum threw a pot at his head, threw a knife at him and then I remember her taking us to the refuge up here. Me mum left with us four boys and we stayed up there all alone with nothing. (Marcus, aged 20)

Sadly, Marcus's mother was ill-equipped to look after herself and the children. She suffered from bipolar disorder and had tried to commit suicide during one severe bout of depression. Overwhelmed and unable to cope, she returned home from the refuge and in Marcus's young eyes his parents were making another go of it.

> A miracle must have happened, because my parents got back together and we started living as a family and then it just crumbled again. I couldn't believe it, man. That really wrecked us, eh, because me mum took off and we didn't see her for years. I still can't get over it to this day. They made a go for it after the big breakup and then they just fell apart again, you know. It's hard trying to keep happy. The whole family collapsed and it hit me. It hit me hard, you know. (Marcus, aged 20)

After their mother left home once again, Marcus's father physically cared for the boys and, in due course, he stopped drinking. However, he continued to beat his children. Marcus was the youngest of four boys in his family. The eldest had already moved out and the others were rarely at home. They were now beyond their father's control. 'All my brothers stuffed up and I was his big last chance. He was really hard on me because he thought I would make it,' Marcus recalled, though this did not stop his father introducing him to marijuana. At one point, he met up with his mother again, but this was not to be a fairytale reunion. She blamed him for the family breakup.

> She was very depressed, but to put all the blame on me for her marriage breaking up, oh mate, hurt, it's not the kind of thing that gets said every day and I haven't seen Mum since that day. I haven't heard from her. She did break my heart and she broke it in a big way. (Marcus, aged 20)

Marcus's future looked bleak; yet even in the depths of fear and despair there was just a dim flicker of hope. Like the majority of the young men from the drop-in centre, he envisaged a possible future involving a job, a home, a car, and a wife and children – in fact, the conventional picture of happy family life. Despite their addictions – and perhaps because of their past – men like Marcus often hanker after their idea of the 'normal'.

> The future scares the shit out of me. It does, man. I wake up and I say to myself, 'what's today gonna bring; a punch in the head, a kick in the teeth,' the first thing that comes into my mind. I think about that every day and it scares the shit out of me, 'cause really I don't know what the future is gonna bring for me. Really, I should be looking at myself and where I'm gonna end up. I can't answer that, I can't answer where I'm gonna end up. I know where I'd like to end up with just a normal family, bringing up your daughter or son. (Marcus, aged 20)

Unhappiness is a family bequest

Marcus's family life was not unique or even particularly unusual among these heroin users from the drop-in centre. In fact, it was the norm. I was repeatedly struck by the fact that these young men (with one exception) had a background in what psychological literature often calls 'dysfunctional families'. However, since this phrase resonates with moral condemnation, I describe them simply as unhealthy and unhappy families. We may call them unhealthy precisely because the participants were unhappy. These families were harmful in the same way that cigarette smoking or the Western diet are damaging. That is, certain social, cultural and psychological conditions give rise to behaviour that causes people to suffer.

As the poet Philip Larkin once famously suggested: 'Your Mum and Dad they fuck you up / They don't mean to but they do'. After many hours devoted to talking to men, to reading books and to examining my own life, I would have to agree. Your mum and dad *can* fuck you up. The conclusion that childhood is the furnace in which the girders of adult emotional life are forged does not surprise me per se. Indeed, this is an increasingly common motif of Western culture. However, the apparently inescapable consequences of family life were starker and stronger than I had expected. There is a very clear, precise and apparently deterministic relationship between these men's experience of parenting and their subsequent emotional health. Wider research evidence supports this conclusion:

> More than 40 international studies have shown that a poor start in life increases the likelihood of poor physical and mental health, a disappointing record at school, low success in the job market, and greater involvement in crime ... in our highly mobile societies where families fragment, money is not the biggest driver in predicting social outcomes. Parenting is.[1]

The young drug users from the drop-in centre told me of disrupted and emotionally distressing family relationships that frequently involved conflict with and between their parents. Most of these families had witnessed divorce and separation. Some now included step-parents, while others were single-parent families, usually centred on mothers. It was, of course, only the stories of the young men to which I had direct access. However, their tales of unhappy parents told me about a chain of emotional injury and deprivation by which wounded parents generated hurt children, who in turn become unskilled parents.

Drug use was a significant factor in the family lives of these young men. One man told me how his alcoholic mother used booze to subdue him while another recounted the occasion on which his father first introduced him to cannabis. We can understand this drug abuse as a marker of the pain parents carry from their own childhood. It is a link in the chain of emotional distress carried on from generation to generation. Unfortunately, these parents were often willing to remove their children from the home while they were still teenagers. Alternatively, the boys ran away from troubled families, becoming rootless at a tender age. All of the young men from the drop-in centre I talked with had spent time as homeless street dwellers.

It was a common feature of these young heroin users that family conflict and violence revolved around fathers and stepfathers. Indeed, a characteristic of the conversations I had with *all* the men was that only a handful spoke affirmatively about their relationship with their fathers. Most men described their connection with male parents as emotionally distant, and some had interactions marked by anger and conflict.

Fathers and sons

'All men are sons and, whether they know it or not, most sons are loyal,' suggests therapist and writer Terrance Real.[2] As a result, sons absorb their father's voice into themselves as the representation of an idealised manhood. Alternatively, since many of our fathers were not emotionally, physically or spiritually available to us, we sons lack the guidance and training that a loving father can offer. The consequence is emptiness at the core of men's being that is filled by overwork, drugs, sex and unsatisfactory relationships.

Fatherhood has become a central theme among researchers concerned with men and masculinity, many of whom describe postwar men as having been emotionally unnourished.[3] Some writers describe this as a 'father-hunger' or 'father-wound' at the heart of contemporary men who mourn lost contact and love with their fathers and express it through anger. Coming to terms with your father, fixing your relationship with him and learning to love the father in oneself are seen as necessary steps towards psychological health.

DISTANT FATHERS

Participants in the 'men's movement' often see their fathers as a particularly significant focus of self-reflection. Douglas (aged 64) felt that his father had not loved him and that this was the root cause of his anger, which in turn had prevented him from loving his son. He said that recognising this had helped him overcome his rage and that, as he ceased trying to control his son, so their relationship improved. This is an archetypical story from the men's movement literature and of my conversations with participants in men's groups. Mike (aged 57) summed up their experience: 'My dad was a hardworking man who I didn't see all that much and he wasn't really there for me emotionally when he was around. I grew up in a house where "I love you" was not a phrase often heard.'

A sense of emotional distance between fathers and sons was also related by many of the business executives with whom I spoke. Ian (a 35-year-old manager with a pharmaceutical company) explained that his relationship with his father was a 'very traditional sort of distant relationship, but I always felt wanted and I guess felt loved, but it was something that we never really discussed or talked about'. This is an emblematic statement. *The Hite Report on the Family*[4] concludes that 'distant' is the predominant emotional tone of most contemporary father–son relationships. Only 18 per cent of boys in the Hite report said that they had a close relationship with their father and 41 per cent of boys (and 32 per cent of girls) described their father as having 'an explosive temper'. Hite suggests that girls' relationships with their fathers can also be troublesome. She reports that girls talk about their fathers in contradictory and extreme ways: he was either wonderful or a monster (38 per cent of girls were very angry with their fathers). However, disengagement and alienation were more clearly features of father–son relationships.

Ian acknowledges that his relationship with his father was 'traditional' and with it the understanding that father–son relationships entail emotional detachment. Though he says that he felt 'wanted' and 'loved', this claim is heavily mitigated by the phrase 'I guess'. The idea that father–son relationships are short on spoken communication is a common feature of male family interactions. This gives rise to a sense of loss that men find hard to adequately express. This is not because men are 'unemotional', but marks the absence of a vocabulary adequate to express this loss. We have not yet thought up enough new metaphors and poetic ways of speaking about emotionally absent fathers to enable us to fully grasp what this means to us.

ANGER AND VIOLENCE

While the majority of men I spoke with described their relationships with their fathers as reserved, the young heroin users told stories not only of detachment but also of conflict and violence.

> He was an angry man and I have no respect for him because of what he has done. One day, a turning point was when I was about five and for some reason I said I didn't like him or something and then he hit me with the belt and then he hit me again and I said 'I hate you' and then he kept on hitting me and I kept on saying 'I hate you'. I didn't want to give in, so I just kept on saying it. And then I'd think to myself, 'Well, I won't do that when I'm older'. That was like a moral decision I was making when I was real young. In a way, I couldn't forgive him for it if he came up and said sorry, because he wasn't on alcohol or drugs or anything. (Matt, aged 19)

Matt's tale of family brutality was not uncommon among the men from the drop-in centre, although the fact that his father was not drinking or using illegal drugs was a rarity. Parental alcohol abuse, especially but not exclusively carried out by fathers, was a picture painted with a sad regularity.

> He was an alcoholic. He used to belt us and he'd be out of control and just worry about the grog and that type of thing. Like, he didn't do anything for us during that time and he neglected us a bit. He got sick of my mum because she used to hound him about the grog. She used to say 'Get off your arse and get a job' and he wouldn't be in it, so he moved out into a hostel for a year and then they got their act together and now they're back together. I felt like I was the black sheep of the family 'cause I was in the middle and whenever there was a fight or something happened at home, I used to get the blame for it and go back to school and not come home for that weekend. So I've hated them for that. (Philip, aged 24)

Alcohol and violence led to the breakup of numerous parental relationships, leaving these young men carrying a sense of loss about their absent dads. Damien poignantly described his relationship with his father:

> My mum left him because of abuse. He said he was gonna keep in contact and everything, but never did and then a couple of years later he showed up on the doorstep with a little puppy dog for me and I thought that was all right, but I never seen him again after that. So I've seen him for about half an hour in 20 years. (Damien, aged 25)

For the sons, the absence of their father under demanding family circumstances commonly led them to experience anger and sometimes depression. Bob described how his sense of loss appeared in the form of anger directed at his mother. Hard-pressed to cope with his increasingly difficult behaviour, she eventually told him to leave the family home.

> She kicked me out because she couldn't handle it anymore, me bringing pot home and things like that and she used to be a churchie; now she's a pisshead, so I did put her through hell. (Bob, aged 22)

Ray (aged 63), a participant in the men's movement, was a father who had resorted to violence. He described 'a silent anger that I unfortunately took out on the kids physically and I felt really bad about that. It was terrible. I am so ashamed. I even hardly talk to him now. I am so ashamed about what I did'. Ray understood his anger and violence to be a manifestation of frustration with his own life and his relationship with his wife in particular. He felt emotionally alienated from her and unable to talk together about sex, relationships and emotion. 'I realise now that I just needed someone to talk to,' he said.

Underlying Ray's difficulties was a long-term depression and a series of panic attacks that originated in an emotionally sterile childhood family: 'The blockage I had from my childhood affected how I was as a father. I am not the only one; a lot of guys say the same thing.' Through the stories of Ray and Marcus, we can see how anger, depression and shame travel like an ancient curse down the generations of a family line. Certainly, the theme of emotionally disturbed and disturbing fathers recurs throughout this book and chimes with my own story.

ALL ABOUT MY FATHER

I have been looking at old family photographs again. Through the images of my father, I touch loss and sadness. He looks like a fragile old man. I recognise the face but not the feeling. He does not appear to be the man I experienced as a child – an aggressive bully who wanted to control me. For much of my life, I have been angry with him. I remember his drunken unpredictability and the menace of brutality that accompanied it. Actual violence was a rarity, but its threat hovered around him like an invisible force field. I felt an ever-present sense of anxiety: what might happen next?

As a boy, I was intimidated by the aggressive anger he directed towards my mother. And somehow I felt obliged to defend her. Family battlelines were drawn up and a slow but bloody war of attrition unfolded. Feeling abandoned by my mother, my father felt wounded by the attention she bestowed upon me, and his resentment was tangible. He certainly took a dislike to the course my life took. While his talents were oriented towards taking apart and building machines, I was attracted to reading and the Humanities. It seemed to me that he didn't like me very much, let alone love me. He was rarely affectionate and often hostile, becoming more inhabited by rage as he got older and more dependent on alcohol. I knew when he had been drinking and was fearful when I smelled the booze on his breath and watched his soul depart from his eyes. One fateful night, at the age of 18, I left home in a hurry when, in another drunken stew, he swayed towards me knife in hand.

For all these reasons, I have found it hard to think of him as my 'dad'. Instead, I have considered him somewhat contemptuously as 'my father'. When he died in hospital, I sat with my mother but did not go in to see his body. 'Who cares?' was what I recklessly told myself. Looking back, I now understand my disdain as a defence against abandonment and grief: that he was not the dad I wished he had been and now he never could be. The sadness I feel when I look at photographs of him is an echo-sound of depthless loss and disappointment.

Yet, he was still my father, and in recent years I have softened my view of him. I now appreciate that he suffered a great deal. His mother lived with poor mental health and he experienced a suffocating childhood.

He was a sensitive man whose aggression, jealousy and drinking were in response to his own fears, insecurities and depression. He craved love and emotional support, as we all do, and did not find it for long enough. I see that we have more in common than I had thought. We have shared feelings of anger, anxiety and depression. When I see that he has suffered as I have, then blame evaporates – and that is a release. I need no longer cling to my anger, mistaking it for a life raft.

It appears that my father and I share a similar biological disposition towards emotional sensitivity, which, when aggravated by childhood experiences, provoked anxiety and depression. I see that we both craved the emotional security that our own families never fully imparted. I know that the path of alcohol and loneliness he trod might so easily have been mine. I took a few steps down that road, but thankfully life offered me another direction. Now I have begun to remember happier times with him when we did things together and he was able to express affection – usually through activity rather than in words. I feel a sense of absence and vulnerability, but I am no longer angry.

A family of emotions: Fear, love and loss

The stories told by the young men from the drop-in centre are so similar that they become almost interchangeable. The precise details of each human tale are different, but the underlying character of the emotional landscapes is alike; namely, parenting that was unable to meet their emotional needs. As children they witnessed conflict between their parents that was often violent and fuelled by drugs and alcohol. They were caught up in conflict with their parents, especially with their fathers and stepfathers, and were sometimes subject to sexual abuse. The outcome was that these were not always easy children or teenagers to live with. Nonetheless, a parental willingness to remove troublesome boys from their homes still comes as a shock. And with it the wheel of emotional injury in families threatens to take another turn.

I drew attention above to the significance of father–son relationships, yet mothers are, of course, equally as important to children's emotional wellbeing (see chapter 5). Indeed, we should not get too entranced discussing the roles of mothers and fathers per se. Rather, our core concern must be with the *quality* of parenting, love and emotional nurturing, whoever gives it or withholds it. The adults involved can vary, but parent–child relationships always involve a significant 'family' of emotions; notably fear (and its cousins anxiety, shame and anger), love (including attachment, connection, joy and compassion) and loss (grief and depression). These core emotions appear repeatedly in the stories of the men we are discussing. The human emotions of fear, love and loss are central to our lives and are connected developmentally in the context of the family.

CHILDHOOD AND EMOTIONAL DEVELOPMENT

Childhood experience shapes adult emotional life in quite fundamental ways. It is a core argument of cognitive psychology and psychoanalysis that the emotional patterns of adult life originate in infancy. After a period in the womb in which all its needs are effortlessly met, a newborn human enters the world as both helpless and needy. This is the condition that an infant has to negotiate with their environment and which constitutes the origin of fear, love and loss.

Most child-development literature suggests that babies are unable to distinguish themselves from other objects (including persons) in the early months of life. Initially, infants experience this condition as omnipotence. However, they soon come to learn that power is an illusion and that they are dependent on others for survival. As infants learn about their dependency, so they develop an increasing sense of self (as differentiated from others) and with it the experience of fear, love and loss.

The processes of feeding and holding are critical to the survival of infants and to their healthy emotional development. Food is necessary for physical growth and a child's demand to be fed is driven by hunger. Yet, feeding is also a primary source of comfort and wellbeing. The holding that accompanies it is an important part of meeting the need for security. The desire to be held and comforted is a common primate heritage and a child's 'failure to thrive' is as much about attention as it is about food.

Yet, neither food nor attention is under the infant's control, which gives rise to a primal fear of abandonment (*loss*) and annihilation. In other words, the experience of *fear* accompanies the infant's realisation that they are dependent on others. A child's awareness of dependency also generates *anger* as they direct fury at those who fail to meet their demands. Further, with the child's realisation that they lack the omnipotence they had assumed, a form of original *shame* arises. As an infant learns that the adult carer returns, so abandonment fears subside, individuation develops and *love* is manifest. However, the figure to whom the infant is attached and to whom they direct love is also the source of *anxiety*. Thus from an early age we are the site of emotional conflicts.[5]

While this primary state of affairs is common to all human beings, it develops uniquely for each of us, with notable consequences for adult emotional life.[6] Family history is clearly related to both emotional wellbeing and patterns of self-destructive behaviour. All of us experience fear, anger, neediness, loss and love during our lives. However, children who have experienced 'good enough' parenting are able to develop a sufficiently secure sense of self to behave in constructive, emotionally intelligent ways as adults. Children who have not had fundamental needs for security met are likely to experience a long-term fear of abandonment.

People who fear childhood rejection face an extended struggle with anxiety, loss and loneliness. They may experience difficulty forming satisfying emotional connections, becoming overly needy and clingy with others. Feeling emotionally vulnerable, they become dependent; and their relationships resemble roller-coaster rides of fear (that one may be left alone), anger (that one has been or might be abandoned), grief (for the loss of connection with another) and depression (as one concludes that abandonment is a result of one's own 'badness'). Of course, some children come through terrible ordeals relatively unscathed, because they possess a remarkable resilience or find alternative ways to be parented.

Actual abandonment and abuse have severe emotional and behavioural consequences. However, so do the less obvious forms of ordinary emotional neglect. Many children are not beaten but nonetheless do not receive sufficient loving attention through being held, soothed and valued. This lack of nurturance often gives rise to adults who carry within them a lifelong sense of emptiness and disconnection. Children who suffer emotional deprivation commonly experience high levels of anxiety and depression in adult life (see chapter 6).

EVERYTHING WENT WRONG

These issues of childhood, parenting and emotional development are clearly demonstrated by the young heroin users. However, similar features were also presented by seven of the 20 men from the Diggers Rest Home. Men who were old enough to be Marcus's grandfather offered stories of childhood families involving alcohol abuse, alienation, separation and violence. Of these seven men, five recounted their own experiences of alcoholism and of the six men who had married, five were subsequently divorced. Eddy's parents did not enjoy a good relationship.

> Grog. Mum unfortunately used to enjoy it too, but not as much as Dad. He was a bit of a playboy. They split up. They separated. Mum went to Perth. I eventually went to Perth myself, but I stayed for a while but we sort of broke up. Everything went wrong in the family. (Eddy, aged 77)

Eddy himself 'lost control of the grog' and soon his wife left him. 'I did the wrong thing. I blame myself. I don't blame her. I blame the grog,' he said. As he said, he valued drinking down at the pub with his mates and playing the piano over all other aspects of his life. Eddy linked some of his problems in later life to the shock of his parents' separation:

> Take away the breakup at home and it would have changed the world. I always wanted them to come back together again. I was awfully hurt. (Eddy, aged 77)

Troubled boys in trouble

Emotional troubles rooted in the home commonly show up as problems at school. The young 'at risk' men from the drop-in centre had experienced 'learning difficulties' and recurrent disciplinary confrontations at school from an early age. They commonly explained this with the phrase 'the teachers didn't like me'. The ambivalence of this claim lies in the fact that they often did struggle with concentration and learning, which led to behaviours that teachers found demanding. Although many teachers will have worked hard to assist these young men as best they could, it is likely that a number of them didn't find the boys very agreeable. Most schools, and especially those located in low-income areas, simply don't have the resources to give disturbed and disturbing children the time and care they need.

> Mainly I got into a lot of trouble at school, and even in primary school I was put out the front of the Principal's office all day to do my work there, because in class I couldn't get along with the teacher or the other kids because I would disturb them or I would make them take their attention off the teacher, which would make the teacher put the attention on me, which would make him cross. I found that I needed more attention than the other kids because I couldn't pick things up as easily as them, because of the ADD. (Stephen, aged 21)

There were common themes to these men's experiences at school: difficulties with concentration, lack of motivation and interest, boredom, truancy, 'disruptive' behaviour that sometimes included violence, marijuana and alcohol abuse (commonly when they truanted, but sometimes while at school) and inevitably suspension and expulsion. This montage of comments from the young men gives a flavour of their feelings and experience of school:

> I was like a problem child and I had never gone to other schools and it was a special school; and then one day they busted me for drinking alcohol in Year 7 and so they suspended me ... Like, I put my mum through hell, I was always getting suspended from school and then I ended up getting expelled from school. It was no good. I never got to learn anything ... In Year 6, when they sent my report card home, it had that I only went for three days in the whole year. I said to my mum, 'Well, you were never around, so what does it matter?' ... I don't know, I didn't find it interesting and the teachers that I had didn't like me and they didn't teach the class properly, like they didn't explain it. Well, I always had food fights, paper fights and just running around ... As soon as I hit high school, that's when I started smoking pot, smoking cigars and

that's when me grades just went down, down, down … I did have a big problem there with the teachers in high school and basically I would just sit there and do nothing. I did get kicked out of school.

And the odd exception:

> It was an escape for me and even when my parents were together I couldn't wait to get to school to get away from them and the fucking dramas. (Alan, aged 20)

Often when boys don't enjoy school they just stop going. One of the outcomes of absence from school – and an ironic side effect of suspension and expulsion – is that they deepen their drug habits. This often follows on from hanging around with older boys and men.

> Because I left school early, all my friends were at school, so I hung around with older people who weren't at school in order to have someone to hang out with, so therefore I was doing things that maybe I shouldn't have been doing. (Paul, aged 23)

I came to appreciate the willingness of these young men to speak openly about themselves. They did not try to hide the troublesome aspects of their lives. However, as a consequence of their limited schooling, they did not generally possess the depth and range of vocabulary deployed by their contemporaries. They were unsurprisingly less skilled with words than the students of the same age that I was teaching at university. The combination of emotional distress and restricted vocabulary led them to be powerfully driven by their feelings. Further, limited schooling radically circumscribed their job prospects, which combined with 'poor' work records and a history of drug use, trapped them in an 'underclass'. They understood that getting work was going to be difficult and this tended to sap them of hope. Without hope, they commonly retreated back into drug use.

Alternative parenting

It is worth considering exceptions to the picture in which fractured families necessarily lead to future emotional difficulties. For example, one of the Diggers and three of the sportsmen demonstrated that a separated and/or emotionally distressed family does not inevitably spawn dire consequences. If parents continue to support their children and conduct themselves lovingly, or if an alternative 'parent' appears on the scene, then children can still grow up relatively happily. For example, in chapter 1 we met 75-year-old Harold, a man with a constructive outlook and a figure of resilience. Well, Harold's parents separated when he was ten; but crucially they continued to share in his upbringing.

> I feel that I had a good relationship with Dad and Mum. They were very careful, each one was careful, not to alienate me from the other. So they had their difficulties but they didn't rub off. I don't feel that they did anything wrong as far as I was concerned. (Harold, aged 75)

Harold worked as a carpenter throughout his life, deriving joy and pleasure from his occupation. He had not suffered from any severe forms of depression, nor was he an alcoholic. In fact, for the most part he was an emotionally sensitive and self-reflective man. Having said that, Harold struggled to sustain relationships. He had been married three times and participated in a couple of other 'serious' relationships. None had lasted and it had been him who left the relationships.

Ashley (aged 23) was a former English under-19s international rugby union player and club-based semi-professional. His parents divorced when he was four, but he spoke of warm and loving parents, including a close relationship with his father, who he loved and respected.

> I felt loved by all my family. Even though my dad had gone away, I still felt that he loved me. It's just the way it was and it was normal for me and Mum never complained. My mum and dad still get on well and nobody ever blamed Dad and now as an older person I can understand how those things happen. (Ashley, aged 23)

Further, Ashley's uncle and grandfather offered him emotionally close male role models who were sporty, with whom he played and arm-wrestled and who he admired. In other words, divorce and a father who is not living in the same house is not necessarily a recipe for emotional discord. Ashley was an intelligent and mature young man.

LOUIS GETS LIFE COACHING

Louis was a 33-year-old African American playing professional basketball in Australia with a championship-winning side in the National Basketball League. He described an emotionally testing childhood in which his father 'didn't know how to show affection' and his mother was frosty and nonchalant. His parents were not happy together (his father had a long-running 'alternative' family) and 'there was always tension in the house'. As a child, Louis 'had no confidence in myself at all'.

Given a discordant family life in a neighbourhood where drugs and gangs were commonplace, we might have expected Louis to be treading the same troubled path as Marcus. However, he was passionate about sport and basketball in particular. He practised all the hours that were available to him and did enough schoolwork to keep him on the right side of teachers, and therefore in the team. He understood that a college scholarship was a route to sporting success and as a youngster he avoided drugs as incompatible with basketball. 'Sport,' he said, 'definitely kept me out of trouble.' Louis's school basketball coach was a particularly important influence on him.

> My high school coach was more of a father to me than my own father. He gave me confidence and once I got confidence my basketball just went swoosh. My school coach was always putting his arm around me and calling me champ – 'hey champ' – and that stuff sticks with you. You start thinking it, you start walking it, then everything changes'. (Louis, aged 33)

Louis's coach didn't only give him support on the basketball court; he also talked to him about how to bear life's ups and downs and encouraged him to attend college.

> I still talk to him and when we talk we talk about, funny enough, everything but basketball. Our relationship started as basketball coach and player, it just evolved, so now we talk about relationships, we talk about politics, we talk about spirituality, we talk about kids, you name it, whatever. Whereas my father, after we finish talking about sports we sit there going ...'. (Louis, aged 33)

In other words, clichéd though it sounds, Louis's basketball coach was a surrogate parent and provided him with much that lucky boys get from their biological fathers. While family love provides the emotional foundations for many of us to go on in life, there are other ways to be 'parented' and develop appropriate esteem and behaviour. For Louis, this came through a sporting mentor.

The bittersweet legacy of family life

I began all my conversations with the many men I talked to by asking about their family of origin. They all had different stories to tell and yet within their distinctions and diversity lay patterns of striking similarity. This finding of sameness within difference is the paradox of all social and cultural investigation, yet it seems particularly strong in relation to the family. The men are all unique and yet I see a strongly determining relationship between the quality of family life as a child and their later capacity for love and emotional wellbeing on the one hand, and conflict, depression and alcoholism on the other.

In this chapter, I have concentrated on the bitter, self-destructive consequences of parenting that is unable to meet a child's emotional needs. In particular, we observed that the torments experienced by young male heroin users could be related, at least in part, to their family of origin. Although less severe in its consequences, this was also the case for many of the other men. I suggested that ineffective parenting and its emotional costs travels down the chain of family connections like a mutant virus. Understanding this enables us to develop forgiveness and compassion for our own parents if we feel hurt by them. It might also suggest that drug addiction is better treated as a psychological and medical issue rather than a criminal one.

Yet, the legacy of family relationships on our future emotional life is not simply a harmful one. Many of us have enduring sweet memories of family outings, a safe pair of arms and a comforting word. The family has it dark corners and terrifying scenes, but it can also light the pathways of joyful living. Your mum and dad may fuck you up, but they can also lay the foundations for happiness and resilience. It is to this theme that we now turn.

Family foundations

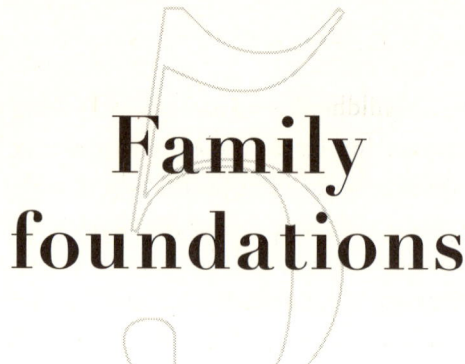

Just as the families of Marcus and his friends were often chaotic and harsh, so a characteristic of the childhood homes of executives was their nurturing constancy. Of course, some families yielded more happy times than others, but the general climate was one of safety, structure and love. There was not a single corporate executive I talked with whose early family environment remotely resembled those of the young heroin users. Not all were idyllic, but none were dangerous; the emotional lives of corporate executives were built on solid foundations.

Graham and Tony strike it lucky

Graham is the 48-year-old chief financial officer of a major fiscal institution. He told me that he had 'a wonderful childhood, a very happy family-centred life'. 'Really, the main thing was time: that they were both very willing to spend a lot of time with us. We were loved and cared for, definitely, in a strong nurturing environment.' A couple of the executives described more thorny family backgrounds than Graham's, including an anxious alcoholic mother prone to violence. However, these more fractious childhood environments were standout exceptions. Mostly, the childhood families of these executives endowed them with the emotional solidity to go out into the world and become socially 'successful' men.

The families of the executives also provided them with significant values that acted as maps in the social universe. For instance, Graham's parents modelled a set of values and behaviours that laid the groundwork for his achievements at school and in business. Throughout our conversation, he described his commitment to what he called the 'protestant ethic'; that is, hard work, personal achievement and family life. Indeed, it was a surprising facet of my conversations that a quarter of these businessmen espoused Christian values.

> My parents had wonderful work ethics. And really have demonstrated to me a very important, the most important, element of family life. Christian values in a general sense. And we try to carry that on with our family. (Graham, aged 48)

Graham's relationship with his father was close and affirmative: 'He was a role model, is the least I can say about him. Hero worship. I aspired to be the sort of man he was. He was always there when I needed him.' Despite this fatherly hero worship, Graham's family life was still 'focused on my mother'. He described her as 'a very loving and caring person who did everything she could for me'. To Graham, his mother was 'probably the closet thing to a saint that I'll ever see on earth'.

Graham's close relationship with his father was unusual even among the executives. More common was the description that Bill (aged 52, a senior educational manager) gave of his dad: 'a standard World War Two father' who worked long hours and was rarely seen by the children. Bill's contact with his father was restricted to weekends, when they interacted through sporting activity. The father–son relationship was a matter of authority and civility more than a deep loving emotional connection. The domestic and child-rearing responsibilities lay with his mother. Indeed, it was largely mothers that provided all the executives with the core of their emotionally supportive home lives.

TONY: MY WONDERFUL MUM

Tony is the 48-year-old chief executive officer of the Australian arm of a major multinational company in the information technology sector. He described his emotional proximity to his mother and a certain distance from his father:

> Mum was very close. Because I was the youngest then I did more with Mum. So Mum and I were very close and I can still remember, you know, when I'd go to bed I'd always get Mum to sit down and put me to bed. I can remember that, I must have been at primary school, but I still remember that. So I was very close to Mum. Dad was, I wouldn't say I wasn't close to Dad, that's not true, but Dad was always, you know, we did sport with him, he was always there, like he used to take me to town when I was in high school and he'd wait for me. So I wasn't as close to Dad. (Tony, aged 48)

This is a rather revealing passage. Three times Tony talks about being 'very close' to his mum, and the memories of being tucked up in bed at night indicate the emotionally intimate character of their relationship. He is reluctant to say that he was not close to his father, but it is significant that this is expressed in the negative. He doesn't want to malign his father, but since he can't honestly claim emotional intimacy, he praises him for the things that he did with and for him. Tony's dad is involved in *doing* things rather more than providing overt emotional closeness, and this in the archetypical male domain of sport. Shared activity such as sport can be men's way of being close with their children and Tony acknowledges this. After all, his dad was 'always there', which is not something we can say about the fathers of the young men from the drop-in centre. However, just being there does not give rise to the same feelings of emotional connection that he experienced with his mother.

This story of a happy, stable mother-centred two-parent family life now has a stereotypical ring about it. It feels more like the ascendant image of the family rather than our actual common experience. Certainly, the majority of people in Western societies no longer live in a conventional 1950s nuclear family; that is, two adult parents and their children living exclusively together under the same roof. Nevertheless, the passage does represent the characteristic pattern among the executives with whom I spoke.

We might feel that these glowing reports of motherhood contain a degree of fantasy and idealisation. Certainly, some of the executives had difficult relationships with their mothers. For example, Derek (a health clinic manager, aged 49) told me his mother was 'a very critical person' and 'an anxious type', characteristics that he felt contributed to his own pessimism and restricted self-esteem. Gordon (aged 48) told me of a mother with 'a bit of a drinking problem, she started arguments and there was some violence. All in all, my relationship with my mother wasn't particularly good.'

The picture is thus more complex than one in which all executives come from happy families with wonderful mothers. Life is always messier and more intricate than such simple truths would allow. Nonetheless, compared with the other groups of men in the book, and the drug-users in particular, most of the executives did have stable, loving family environments as children in which mothers played the key nurturing role.

Not only do mother–child relationships lay the foundations for later life, but also positions of corporate power rely on the practical and emotional support given by women: 'I don't think I could do it without having a kind of stable family life you know, it's been very good' (Tony, aged 48). This is consistent with a view that the psychological dynamics of the modern family position boys as independent adventurers geared to the external world. Boys are forged psychologically to want to explore and 'master' their exterior environment.[1] It is within our family that we first stitch the key values modelled to us by our parents to a feeling of emotional security and become bonded to cultural ideas, whose illusory solidity makes us feel safe.

Gerard: The value of success

Gerard, who we met in chapter 1, was a 36-year-old senior executive with a major telecommunications company with responsibility for their relations with government. He told me: 'The routine that I saw my parents set was one of steady, solid work and it was a house with a lot of books and so on.' Both Gerard's parents worked full-time and after the family meal his father, a professor, would 'go and work for two or three hours each night'. The value that Gerard's parents ascribed to work was thus apparent to him.

As a child, Gerard did not feel emotionally close to his father, who enacted the somewhat remote work-oriented man. However, these feelings did not necessarily reflect lack of contact or care, since his father 'allocated a lot of time to me ... coaching me to get a scholarship'. As Gerard acknowledged, 'the models were there to follow'. And follow them he did, with achievements at private school and university preceding a career as a lawyer, advisor to a government minister and high-powered corporate executive.

It is not particularly surprising that the commitment to worldly success nurtured in Gerard's family manifested in educational accomplishment. Indeed, all but one of the executives attended university, and although a couple paused for a moment of youthful rebelliousness, they too got there in the end. These executives got on the achievement train at primary school and took the ride all the way to the top station. Nonetheless, the majority of these men were not the children of the very rich (only one fitted that mould), but rather of middle-class professionals (doctors, teachers, farmers, businessmen, managers, and so on), with five hailing from more working-class families. Consequently, they had to study in order to meet their aspirations and, for the most part, they enjoyed school.

> For me, school was quite a pleasurable experience. I was one of those kind of irritating sort of swotting children who liked school. I did very well academically at school. I worked very very hard. I was involved in quite a few extracurricular activities, debating I did lot of. I was editor of the school magazine. I played a lot of sport, not very well but I participated. I was a prefect, so I was kind of, it was all part of the whole, you know, totally buying into the whole experience and I enjoyed it. I enjoyed school. (Gerard, aged 36)

Achievement at school often requires a degree of 'emotional intelligence' (EI). As popularised by Daniel Goleman[2], EI constitutes a basic requirement for the effective use of intellectual intelligence (IQ). It allows us to judge the situation we are in and to act appropriately. When we act with emotional intelligence, we are not swept away by our immediate feelings but are able to pause, reflect and act more skilfully. Compared to the young men from the drop-in centre, these executives showed higher levels of emotional intelligence developed as a child (but see chapter 8 for the emotional limitations of executives). The young drug users brought unhappy feelings and wavering concentration to school, which led them into conflict with teachers. In contrast, the executives-in-making were developing a calm focus and deference to authority that underpinned 'success' in the education system and other organisational environments.

THINKING EMOTION

The emphasis that the executives give to socially sanctioned achievement is a reflection of their emotionally charged 'family values'. In the furnace of childhood, we forge a connection between our values and emotions that lies at the heart of who we think we are. For example, the character of men like Gerard involves emotional identification with a particular idea of success. It is the way executives think about themselves that is at the core of their emotional lives and these executives are emotionally attached to financial and organisational achievement at work. Their happiness is fused to such thoughts as 'I am a success' and 'I have done well'. Indeed, how we *think* is central to all our emotional lives.

Doubtless there is a hard-wired component to emotion that has been fashioned by our evolutionarily needs. But we also know that cognition plays a central role in human feelings. The idea of cognition simply refers to 'information processing' by the brain, with verbal thinking being a particularly significant human dimension. Philosopher Martha Nussbaum[3] argues persuasively that an emotion is constituted by judgments we make in relation to objects that are of importance to our world and wellbeing. In other words, emotions involve cognitive judgments about value. They are suffused with intelligence that appraises external objects as salient to our wellbeing. For example, the thinking of executives like Gerard and Tony include judgments that a highly paid job is a sign of success and that public achievement is necessary to their happiness.

Physiological feelings are intrinsic to cognition, so all thinking has an affective dimension. For example, the thought 'I am in danger' entails bodily responses such as a speeding heart and sweaty palms that we name as 'fear' or 'anger'. This naming can set off further emotional responses. At the feet of their parents, executives learnt to value social success and acquired the means to attain it. When they receive the rewards of achievement, they are able to think 'I have done well' and conclude that 'I am a good person'. These thoughts are accompanied by feelings of self-worth and wellbeing. However, any hint of failure may take them down the reverse spiral towards depression (see chapter 6). The young heroin users we encountered entered this space long ago. The circumstances of their family lives led them to thoughts such as 'I am worthless', 'I will never amount to anything' and 'It's all my fault'. Such thoughts are the cognitive foundation of hopelessness and despair.

American psychologist Martin Seligman[4] has played an important role in demonstrating the significance of thinking styles to emotion through his investigation of optimism and pessimism. He explores the way in which a gloomy worldview constituted by a learnt vocabulary of pessimism (entailing thoughts such as 'Things always go wrong for me') underpins an array of 'affective disorders'. He cites evidence to suggest that in Western culture pessimistic scripts are learnt more commonly from mothers than from fathers. Acquiring the language of pessimism or optimism changes our biochemistry. For example, Seligman provides evidence that pessimistic thinking depletes the immune system, while optimism boosts it. The way we think can alter the biochemistry of the brain, so that childhood experience can have lifelong psychobiological consequences.

The value of attachment

There are alternative ways to explain children's development towards emotional maturity. However, a theme I found to be recurrent within the literature and convincing in its arguments concerns the importance of childhood emotional 'attachments' to their subsequent wellbeing. Attachment is the strong emotional connection that arises between infant and caregiver, and which provides the child with emotional security. We more commonly call this love.

In our ancestral past, when small children were in constant danger of being eaten by a predator, remaining close to adults protected them from danger. Human beings who had strong attachment drives were more likely to survive than those who did not. Consequently, as time passed, a compulsion to attach became more strongly embedded in the human gene pool. Because of the selective advantages conferred by staying close to parents, an attachment system is part of our primate evolutionary endowment and is encoded in the human nervous system. The very nature of human beings compels infants to seek attachment with their caregiver.

Through actions like smiling and crying, a young child aims to bring adult attachment figures such as their mother close to them. Rooting, grasping, sucking, following, approaching and clinging are all ways by which an infant actively seeks proximity and contact with their carers.[5] Accordingly, after about six months, infants have become attached to familiar people who have responded to their need for physical care and mental stimulation.

However, human beings also need to go out into the world to find food and mates, so soon a new compulsion becomes activated urging us to explore our external world. Since exploration is antithetical to remaining close at hand, the relationship between infant and mother entails negotiating a balance between attachment and adventure. Children check the availability and attentiveness of the caregiver in a permanent monitoring activity. Following each reassurance, the child wanders off to play; after a while, they return, and so on. In this pattern, a baby uses their mother as a secure base to which they may return. When a child feels secure, they may confidently explore their surroundings. When a child feels insecure, they may return to their secure base.

The patterns of our emotional life are shaped by the formation, maintenance, disruption or renewal of attachment relationships, which constitute an emotional spectrum of safety and anxiety. When an infant seeks and receives protection, reassurance and comfort, feelings of security and confidence arise. Self-assured exploration is possible because of the love, support and availability of the caregiver. Insecure patterns of emotional life develop when our need for attachment and security is met by rejection, inconsistency or threat, which leaves a child apprehensive and fretful. Will she come back? What will happen to me? The infant who has been routinely rejected is likely to avoid subsequent attachment for fear of being rejected once again. The child whose mother has sometimes responded with warmth and at other times with apparent rejection will seek attachment, but will be remain riven by anxiety.

The centrality of love to human wellbeing is at the heart of this discussion. Our early parent–child relationships are prototypes of later love relationships. It is through them that we build up our broad outlook on the world. For example, when our mothers leave us but consistently return, we are able to expand our confidence in other people. Conversely, if we suspect that we have been abandoned, we become anxious about our world. From these early experiences, we build up a set of assumptions about how *all* close relationships operate. These cognitive patterns are called 'working models' and act as guides to behaviour and relationships. They are relatively stable constructs that operate outside awareness. They are 'burned' into the brain through the strengthening of repeatedly used synaptic connection, though they remain open to revision.

If an attachment figure acknowledges an infant's need for comfort and protection while simultaneously respecting the necessity for independent exploration, the child is likely to develop an internal working model of the 'self' as valued and reliable. The child is able to go out into the world with confidence and is able to love others because he or she values himself or herself. Broadly speaking, the sportsmen we met in chapter 2 who maintained a sense of emotional balance experienced this style of relationship. For example, Jeff the Olympic athlete talked about the 'tremendous love' he felt from his mother, and rugby league star Craig described the 'great relationship' he had with his parents. It was also the mode of family life that executives like 50-year-old Peter told me about.

> I remember my childhood with great affection. You know, I always felt my mum and dad loved me and supported me. Okay, so I got into trouble sometimes, who doesn't, but it always passed and they were always there ... They encouraged me at school and you know kept on

motivating me. I don't think they were that thrilled by my choice of career, Mum you know was a bit arty and stuff, but they never complained and they always just said how proud they were. (Peter, aged 50, managing director of a retail company)

Conversely, if a parent has frequently rejected (or is *felt* to have rejected) an infant's bids for either comfort or independence, the child is likely to construct an internal working model of self as unworthy and incompetent. A child's most common reaction in the face of family confusion is to take responsibility for the parent in order to preserve the emotional attachment. In a desperate attempt to maintain the sanctuary of being cared for by competent adults, children will reproach themselves rather than their parents so that a powerful sense of personal shame is built into their character.[6]

Jake (see chapter 1) was a young unemployed former heroin user who suffered from depression and periodically lived on the streets. He was born into a family in which drugs and violence were commonplace. He lost contact with his father at a very early age and suffered from intense feelings of abandonment.

> Well what would happen was that something would happen like my mum would tell me off or something and I would just go down down. Heavy like and all these thoughts would come to me and these horrific feelings and it would go on for days and I couldn't even remember why I was pissed off any more. It started with a reason, you know, there was some reason why I felt down but I couldn't remember it anymore. (Jake, aged 23)

Emotional life is not as stark or straightforward as the contrast between Peter and Jake might suggest. We are not simply securely attached or anxiously attached. These are merely the extreme points of a messier continuum in which we experience degrees of safety and anxiety. As I explored my own depression, I was initially baffled by the fact that, although my family life had its challenges, I was never abused like Jake. I couldn't see what there was in my relationship with my mother that could have contributed to my own recurrent feelings of anxiety, which I now see were an ever-present feature of my childhood.

My mother's face

My childhood is now uncertain, impossible to locate with any exactness. I know there can be no absolute truths to be found here. Yet, just like the invisible mechanics of quantum physics, the consequences of forces and actions remain. My mother must have her part in my life story. Perhaps unfairly, I have examined my family for the seeds of depression more than those of joy. My mother certainly looked after me physically. I was fed and clothed, taken on holidays, and looked after well enough. I know that she cared for me night and day for two years when I was a sick baby. In fact, I don't recall any specific childhood trauma with her. But it's what I don't remember, an absence, that has left its mark, I think. It is traced on her face. In almost any family photograph, my mother does not smile. Her face is worried and furrowed, downtrodden and pained, without humour or lightness of touch. She is not there. The *lack* was passed on: the lack of smiles, the lack of cuddles, the lack of touch and the lack of connection.

She had her reasons, her place in the causal chain of fucked-up-ness. My mother had hard times: her father died when she was ten, she took on family responsibilities at a young age, a man she loved was killed in the Second World War, and her husband became an alcoholic. She tried to shut out the pain as we all do. To escape, she took her eyes and her mind off somewhere else. Suddenly, it dawns on me. A revelation. My mother was often depressed. We have that in common. Suddenly, I feel empathy and sadness for her. My mother is not a bad person, a mean person or a hurtful person. She is a person who has also been hurt. The effects of depressed mothers on their children can be thus: anxious attachment, neediness, disassociation, depression, drug and alcohol dependency and relationship difficulties.

I don't doubt that my mother loved me. She even spoiled me. I was often favoured over her husband. But she wanted my support in return. It was a part of the family politics. She wanted me to shine for her. And I did try to please her, to make her proud. But nothing is ever quite good enough for Mum (or for me). There is always a darkening cloud to be found in the blue sky and the glittering prize so often turns out to be base metal. My mother loved me and cared for me, but she never told me so. I don't remember an occasion in which she said: 'I love you'. Strangely, I have quite warm memories of childhood illnesses, because when I was sick she comforted me. On other occasions, my mother's love wouldn't quite translate to human warmth. I wanted the touch of her hand, the warmth of her body and a word of love. I wanted the embrace of unconditional love that encircles the world and makes it possible to carry on. I always felt myself to be wanting.

The purpose of exploring the past is to understand and to forgive. I do not blame my mother for anything in my life. She did the best she could in difficult times. She had her own history and her own demons. There is nothing to reproach her for: it all lies in the family tree of cause and effect. The child in the parent breeds the parent in the child and the distinction between good and bad collapses. Blameless children fucked over by blameless parents make blame no longer the issue. Then there are also the achievements of my life: the intellectual ability, the play of words, books, the capacity to love and the joy. Of these too she partakes.

Childhood attachment and adult behaviour

We have seen that a number of the young men from the drop-in centre had an alcohol-abusing parent, as did I. Research[7] tells us that adult men who have an alcoholic parent are more likely to be fearful and themselves suffer from alcoholism. Several studies have found associations between childhood insecurity and adult anxiety, depression and alcohol abuse. Further, a characteristic of men classified with 'ambivalent attachment' is the feeling that their fathers were unfair to them. As we have seen, the drug users had more hostile relationships with their fathers than did the executives or, more strikingly, the sportsmen (see chapter 2).

The degree of childhood security that we achieve through loving relationships with our parents is a significant factor in whether we are ourselves able to develop dependable and loving adult relationships. The relationships that the executives built with their wives and children were by no means models of perfection (see chapter 9), but most of them could sustain partnerships. The men from the drop-in centre, however, had much more difficulty establishing and developing relationships of any sort. Sexual partnerships tended to be short-term affairs and most of the men were single. Nonetheless, the desire to maintain a relationship with a girlfriend was the single most powerful motivation for them to relinquish drug use (see chapter 11).

Seventy-eight per cent of a sample of men in distressed marriages felt insecure, with research[8] telling us that anxious people report higher levels of relationship breakups. Further, people who classified themselves as ambivalently attached describe high intensity of emotion and obsession across a whole range of life experiences, including sexual attraction, jealousy, and desire for union. Separation anxiety and severe discord in the family of origin also predict the use of controlling behaviours to maintain proximity to a partner. Research demonstrates that people who classify themselves as ambivalently attached also report feeling the loneliest.

These findings suggest that insecure attachment as a child gives rise to emotional troubles in adulthood, whereas positive educational achievement and happy moods are supported by safe family backgrounds. Children who are securely attached tend to be more emotionally stable and resilient as adults. This appears to be the case for most of the sportsmen we met in chapter 2 and for the majority of the executives.

The strong connection between class, family life and later emotional development is illustrated by the striking contrast between young heroin users and executives. My conversations with older ex-servicemen from the rest home confirmed the emotional significance of childhood experiences within the same age and class cohort.

Generations

The Diggers were of the generation that fathered the executives. They are also the metaphoric grandparents of the sportsmen and the homeless youngsters. Seven of these 20 elderly men told me childhood family stories involving alcohol abuse, distant relationships, separation and violence (see chapter 4). By contrast, ten of them described their early family life as close, loving and supportive. Their subsequent life stories did not contain any mention of depression or alcoholism and of the nine who had married, only one had been divorced.

VICTOR: THE BEST MUM AND DAD YOU COULD HAVE

Victor spent a lifetime of hard manual work on the trawlers and timber mills. His life was by no means easy, but he had no history of depression or alcohol abuse. He didn't drink and had sustained a loving 40-year marriage. He had also maintained good relationships with his children, who regularly visited him with a brood of cheerful grandkids in tow. He described his marriage and children as forming 'a very happy family'. Crucially, this was also the case for his parents.

> I had a good relationship with my mother and my father. No man or woman could ever get a better mother and father than I had. I was loved by them. They loved me and I loved them. (Victor, aged 75)

When I asked him about any sorrow in his life (amidst the series of positive stories he told), he described his greatest loss as the death of his parents. 'Well, I did have two sadnesses really, which I must admit. First, I lost my mother; that really hurt me. Secondly, I lost my father.' His father died at the age of 91, while his mother was 84.

> *Victor:* I don't look for bad things. Bad things spoil your life. You've got to look for the good things in life.
> *Interviewer:* Where do you think you learnt that?
> *Victor:* Family life. Mum and Dad, they were good people.

THE CHRISTIAN FAMILY

It is interesting that half of the Diggers who told me about contented childhoods had an active Christian faith that was rooted in their family. This was also the case for 25 per cent of the executives. There is some evidence (see chapter 11) that religious beliefs are correlated with a more contented outlook on life. This is probably connected with the sense of purpose that religion carries along with the social connections that it enhances. For example, in chapter 1 Edward (aged 89) described himself as having 'a personal relationship with our Lord' that formed the bedrock for his emotional survival. As he told me: 'Christianity has been a help to me, it has strengthened my resolve to go and do the right things ... I would say that I have lived a contented life believing in Jesus Christ.' Edward's Christian faith helped him through 'tough times' that included a Japanese POW camp, the Burma Railway and the death of his two much-loved wives.

Stan's family hailed from a mining village around Durham in the north-east of England. This is a hardworking and often hard-drinking male-dominated community, and his father was frequently at work and absent from the home. However, the family were not drinkers; rather, they belonged to that tradition of Methodist churchgoers which formed the backbone of English Christian socialism. Stan had a relatively austere but loving childhood in which he felt cherished and cared for.

> I don't remember much about my father, but I do remember him as a kind man though he wasn't there much. There was a lot of hardships, you know, in those days. It was tough times and we struggled as a family from one day to the next. But I never felt anything but love from my mother. She was a believer, you know, a Christian, and she passed that on to all of us kids. (Stan, aged 89)

After his family migrated to Australia, the physical dimensions of Stan's life were challenging, but he had a strength of character that enabled him to face up to all that life offered: 'You knew that you'd have hardships no matter, so you'd just have a happy life as you went along. There was no concern for anything else, no good lying down saying, "Oh, what have I got to be happy for?".' He didn't drink or smoke and described himself as a 'churchman above all'.

Temperament and personality

The association between childhood family experiences and later emotional strategies is robust and persuasive. Nevertheless, the story is more complex than a simple black-and-white correlation between family background and depression or alcoholism. Some men face challenging childhoods but come through relatively unscathed, while ostensibly less severe forms of trauma trouble others greatly.

Maurice (the 37-year-old marketing manager of a pharmaceutical company) described his mother as 'a very strong-willed and domineering woman. I love her dearly but, no, that's not the right word. I wouldn't choose her as a friend'. This is not exactly a glowing report of motherly love, but Maurice was a relatively stable and successful executive – though it is true to say that he was strongly driven to the point of ruthless obsession. In contrast, Ricky (aged 22) described his parents as supportive and told me that he had experienced a happy childhood. He could find no explanation for his own heroin addiction other than his circle of friends and his own choices. Heroin addiction is not always or simply a matter of family-originated emotional pain.

Developmental psychology can leave the impression that we are all hostages to an inevitable blueprint of emotional life rooted in childhood experience. Yet, modes of emotional deprivation or support diverge and the consequences of childhood experience work themselves out differently. For some the adult manifestations of childhood emotional neglect are withdrawal and timidity, while for others it is exhibited through anger and aggression. Certain individuals demonstrate high levels of resilience in overcoming 'difficult' childhoods, while others whose family life has involved far less obvious emotional difficulties fail to thrive. The seeds planted at childhood grow differently in varying social and cultural soils.

No doubt, any adequate explanation for our divergent responses to suffering depends on the details of individual lives, but in general terms they can be explored through the concepts of 'temperament' and 'personality'. Psychologists describe our broad genetically based orientations towards being introvert/extrovert, passive/aggressive, anxious/fearless, emotionally flat/intense, sensitive/invulnerable, and so on, as our temperament. However, that temperament is worked over for each of us by social forces and manifested in quite specific ways as our personality. A safe and nurturing family environment can support a temperamentally shy child so that they become relatively outgoing. A comparatively buoyant and resilient child can be beaten down by sufficient trauma.

Particular combinations of temperament and personality traits give rise to distinct strategies for dealing with emotional discontent. Psychologists Jeffery Young and Janet Klosko[9] describe surrender (maintenance), escape (avoidance) and counterattack (compensation) as different emotional styles for coping with similar feelings. Take, for example, the sense that one is unloved and inadequate. A surrender response accepts that we are defective and interprets a variety of situations as confirming this view. Surrender repeats and extends our childhood experiences. If we feel inadequate and unloved as a child and adopt the surrender strategy, depression is the likely outcome. I must say that my own bouts of depression have been accompanied by a sense of 'giving up', which does have its attractions: no need to struggle any more; the world will have its way.

Some of us surrender into depression, but others adopt strategies of escape by which they attempt to cover over and avoid emotional difficulties. Indeed, they may seek to avoid feeling at all. Alcoholism and other forms of drug abuse are common escape strategies, as is an obsession with work and the avoidance of intimacy in relationships. Maurice (above) was not depressed, but he was a workaholic, and most of the young men from the drop-in centre were using drugs as a way of escaping emotional distress.

Compensatory or counterattacking strategies of emotional management try to make up for emotional anguish and loss by staging the opposite of child experience. In order to overcome feelings of helplessness and worthlessness, one makes oneself feel superior and important; for example, through criticising and devaluing others or by attracting praise through high levels of public achievement. Gordon (above) was an executive who had a testing relationship with his alcoholic and violent mother. He did not talk about depression, but he did recount his tendency towards anger and a highly critical attitude towards others.

The big picture

Surrender, escape and counterattack are 'archetypical' strategies and we should expect any given individual to display a range of them. I have sometimes surrendered into depression, occasionally sought escape through alcohol or work and noticed in myself a marked tendency to counterattack male authority figures. However, in order to connect particular individuals with wider trends in society some generalisation is warranted.

The big picture painted in chapter 4 concerned the way in which men exhibit the emotional consequences of chaotic and/or insecure childhood families. There was a particular focus on the significance of fathering, though I do not wish to suggest that they are solely responsible for emotional disturbance. By contrast, in this chapter we have seen how supportive and secure family environments lay the groundwork for later emotional intelligence. Without implying that they are alone responsible for emotional security, there was a particular focus on the role of mothers.

Executives and professional sportsmen manifested emotional confidence rooted in family life more often than other groups of men. That is, a secure family foundation enabled them to become successful in their chosen fields. The varied pattern of safety and anxiety experienced by the older Diggers demonstrated the significance of early family experiences within the same working-class and age-related cohort.

Overall, the level of secure emotional attachment achieved as a child is a major predictor of the way in which we handle life's vicissitudes. Further, the crucible of family life helps us to forge an emotional bond with the values we have learnt. Needless to say, this is only a rough guide to the formation of our emotional lives. There are men who are able to overcome the influence of childhood traumas and there are others who, despite apparently secure and supportive childhoods, become drug users or suffer from depression. In any case, the family is a significant point of departure, both genetically and culturally, for any explanation of the current epidemic of depression in Western societies. It is to this issue as it impacts men that we now turn in chapter 6.

Men and depression

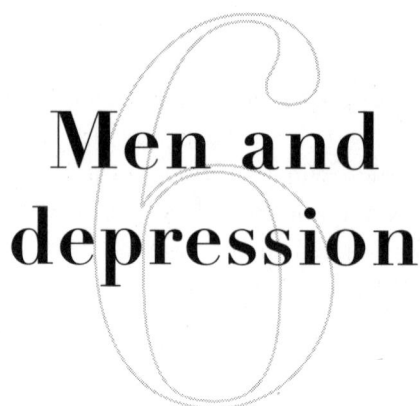

During the spring of 1990, I suffered from severe and repeated headaches simulating a nine-inch nail driven into my head. The throbbing fluctuated over many months, but was particularly severe at weekends – exactly when I thought it ought to disappear, since work-related stress was the official explanation. I medicated myself with exercise and alcohol, achieving a degree of short-term relief; but still I grew increasingly unhappy. Work was a source of anxiety, while increasing marital conflict marked my home life. One day, overwhelmed by a feeling of intense hopelessness, I burst into tears. This time, a six-month course of antidepressants followed and the mood lifted. My doctor diagnosed a mild bout of depression, but issued the ominous warning that we could not know if the experience would repeat itself.

A change of jobs followed and life seemed to be looking up. However, my marriage continued to deteriorate and I felt abandoned. My wife and I entered into relationship counselling, but the disintegration continued and eventually I left the marriage. My moods swung radically from high to low, from hope to despair. I felt relieved that an unhappy marriage was ended, but was overwhelmed with guilt and shame in relation to my children whom I have always loved. And so began a decade-long series of depressive bouts that took me to the precipice. Of course, I am only one of many men and women who have experienced depression in contemporary society; in fact, we are witnessing an epidemic.

The rise and rise of depression

Psychologist Martin Seligman points to a ten-fold increase in the incidence of depression in the West since the First World War. At this very moment, there are nearly 19 million Americans and 1 million Australians who are depressed. Some one in four women and one in six men will suffer from depression during their lives, but 80 per cent will not receive treatment.[1] A survey of six European countries reports that 17 per cent of the population had experienced depression in the previous six months.[2]

Studies confirm that 10 per cent of the US population has experienced major depression in the past year and 20–25 per cent of women and 7–12 per cent of men will suffer from clinical depression in a lifetime. Depression is a condition prone to relapse, and at least 50 per cent of those who recover from an initial episode of depression will have at least one other occurrence. People with a history of two or more depressive episodes have a 70–80 per cent likelihood of repetition.[3]

Australia now ranks third in the world per capita prescription rates for antidepressants after Sweden and France, closely followed by the United States, Canada, the United Kingdom, Germany and Italy. More that 8 million prescriptions for antidepressants were written in Australia in 1998, an increase of 3 million since 1990. Depression has risen from the tenth most common problem seen by GPs to the fourth. One in 16 Australians currently meet the criteria for clinical depression and one in five Australians suffer from a form of mental illness at some point in their lives.

Figures suggest that depression is twice as prevalent among women as among men. However, this difference may be explained by men's notorious reluctance to seek treatment. Men are also more likely to mask depression with drugs and alcohol than women, with some 11 per cent of men compared to 4.5 per cent of women treated for substance abuse.[4] Men are also more likely to commit suicide than women and account for 80 per cent of such deaths. It is estimated that 70 per cent of people who kill themselves are suffering from depression.[5]

Australian suicide rates have increased by 24 per cent since the middle of the 19th century and have become the second highest in the world. Suicide rates among young men aged 15–29 have increased from 5.8 per 100 000 in 1964 to 17.8 per 100 000 in 1990[6], rising further to 27.3 per 100 000 by 1996.[7] Over the last 30 years, the suicide rate among the 15–24-year-olds has tripled.[8] In 1999, two out of five deaths among men in the 25–39 age group were attributable to suicide and another 25 per cent to accidental poisoning, mainly from alcohol or drugs. Almost as many young men died from transport accidents, some of which will have been suicides.

THE EXPERIENCE OF DEPRESSION

The psychiatric diagnostic manual *DSM-IV* describes clinical depression as a mood disorder marked by persistent dejected mood, loss of interest in normal daily activities, poor sleeping patterns, loss of appetite, impaired concentration, and feelings of hopelessness and worthlessness. A diagnosis of major depression is given when a number of these conditions are present for at least two weeks and interfere with daily life. Depression, which is often accompanied by anxiety, may be masked from self-awareness, showing up as problematic behaviour such as alcohol and drug abuse.

Psychologist Dorothy Rowe reports that, when asked to paint a mental picture of depression, people imagine standing alone in a fog, trudging across empty landscapes, being pressed down by a weight, wrapped in a shroud or trapped in a cage: 'But, however the image is expressed, all the images have one thing in common. The person is enduring a terrible isolation. You are alone in a prison'.[9]

A popular self-help book[10] lists the following more specific signs of depression.

Symptoms of depression

Mood

Feeling sad, moody or dispirited

Feeling irritable and unable to cope

Feeling guilty and blaming yourself

Feeling dead or numb emotionally

Dreading everyday activities

Behaviour

Lack of energy and motivation

Sluggishness and a decrease in activities

Weepiness and agitation

Social withdrawal or dependency on people

Increased use of drugs and alcohol

Thinking

Being overly self-critical

Blaming yourself for doing dreadful things

Negative expectations about the future

Imagining others are putting you down

Thinking of suicide and planning it

Physical health

Loss of appetite and weight loss

Overeating or food cravings

Disturbed sleep patterns

Loss of interest in sexual activities

Feeling physically ill

The roots of depression

THE EVOLUTIONARY INFLUENCE

From an evolutionary perspective, emotions emerged because they helped our ancestors to solve the problems of survival. Fear makes us run from danger, anger prompts us to defend ourselves, sexuality is necessary for reproduction and love helps us care for one another. Research suggests that the separate symptoms of depression and anxiety are 33–46 per cent heritable. The co-inheritance of the two conditions is 99 per cent.[11] Some genetic scientists contend that a predisposition towards depression is associated with the gene TH5.

Evolutionary psychology does not reduce emotions to simple genetic determination but is concerned with evolved cognitive mechanisms; that is, templates for human thinking and behaviour that appear because they contain successful solutions to human problems. Depression may have originated in 'surrender' behaviour (Involuntary Defeat Strategy – IDS), such as making oneself look small and unthreatening by curling up in a ball. The adaptive value of this behaviour was to accept defeat, thereby reducing the likelihood of further conflict and real injury.[12]

THE CULTURAL INFLUENCE

Within our prehistoric cave community, an IDS could have been usefully triggered by a confrontation with the most powerful male in the tribe. Today, it may be set off by office politics, the need to meet work deadlines or by a romantic rebuff. Above all, our own internal self-critical thought processes can activate a strategy that is no longer appropriate or useful in contemporary life. A cognitive mechanism that once had adaptive value may now be an impediment. In particular, people who suffer from depression may have a slow IDS recovery process.

The rise of depression in the Western world to epidemic proportions cannot be attributed to genetics *alone* for the time scales involved are radically different. The evolution of genetic capacities takes thousands of years, whereas our steep rise in depression has occurred over the last 50 years. Contemporary social conditions have increasingly triggered biochemical proclivities and emotional responses that may have been germane for our ancestors but which are now destructive.

Cultural factors contributing to the growth of depression include rising expectations of material living standards, leading to work-related stress. The pursuit of wealth and its associated consumption also generates a speed-up in daily life, giving us little time to 'stop and smell the roses'. As our growing individualism disrupts family structures and weakens community support networks, our culture is simultaneously less able to sustain meaning systems that give purpose and direction to life.

A failure to love

Depression has both long-term evolutionary origins and more recent cultural causes. Alongside these large-scale explanations, we need to explore the details of individual experience in order to grasp the nature of depression. According to psychologist Dorothy Rowe, the prison house of depression is built by acquiring interlinked patterns of thought, including: No matter how good and nice I appear to be, I am really bad, evil and valueless. I am unacceptable to myself and to others. People are such that I must fear, hate and envy them. Life is terrible and death is worse. Only bad things happened to me in the past and only bad things will happen to me in the future. It is wrong to get angry and I must never forgive anyone, least of all myself.

At the heart of depression is the thought 'I am not good enough', an idea that first appears during childhood. Children who suffer varying degrees of trauma commonly take on board feelings of worthlessness and shame (see chapters 4 and 5).[13] For example, the young men from the drop-in centre told tales of loss and insecure family attachments. These were stories about a failure to love and its consequences. A number of the young men had made suicide attempts and Stephen was tragically successful. Above all, the use of drugs as a means to numb emotional pain is suggestive of covert depression among *all* these young men.

BEN: HEROIN IS MY ANTIDEPRESSANT

Ben (aged 23) described himself as 'a waste of space on this earth' and had made a number of suicide attempts. He told me: 'I hate life, I hate the world. Heroin is my antidepressant.' Ben was raised amidst 'high-rises, drugs and chaos' with parents who 'couldn't help us help ourselves'. His father was a violent multiple-drug user and dealer who frightened Ben and his mother. She was an alcoholic – 'the drunken bitch' – who left the family home when Ben was 13: 'She went tenpin bowling and never came back.' He felt that he had not recovered from the pain of her disappearance and told me about the anger he felt towards his parents, and women in general.

> *Interviewer:* What is the appeal of heroin, then?
> *Ben:* Numbness. I saw my parents using things to escape, so it was an escape.
> *Interviewer:* Do you get depressed?

> **Ben:** Oh yeah, very depressed, as long as I can remember. I am very angry, I have a lot of anger in me. Relationships are no good for me. Women, ugh. The way my mum and my father were. I'm a lot like my father in that sense. My mother pissed him off and he would go off his head and he would cause havoc.
> **Interviewer:** Can you describe what it's like when you feel depressed?
> **Ben:** I never thought I could feel hurt in my heart, but I do feel hurt in my heart, like a real bad anxiety. I don't know how to explain it.

Ben said that loneliness was a major feature of his life. From an early age, he was left to fend for himself amid the 'dramas with my family'. He expressed distrust of relationships with women and felt safer with his mates. However, he no longer had many close friends because they were either dead or in jail (where he had also spent time). Ben was caught in a paradox. On the one hand, 'I feel that I've got no trust for nobody, I don't trust anybody.' But on the other hand, he described himself as forming 'co-dependent' (his word) relationships with women because 'I need to be needed, I'm a very lonely person'. And there is nothing lonelier than depression.

Ben's life story is stark and could be read as exceptional because he is living in a marginalised world. Nonetheless, anxiety, depression and anger were widespread among all the men I spoke with. In each group, I encountered participants who talked about their depression and our culture now contains a powerful stream of despondent men. My own experience was not as extreme or traumatic as Ben's. Nonetheless, it suggests that a child can be deeply distressed by the apparently insignificant experience of a depressed mother's illegible face.

My melancholy family

I will never know with certainty the causes of my anxiety and depression. However, I can put forward a plausible explanation based on contemporary biological and psychological insights. For example, it is widely held that anxiety and depression 'runs in families'. My paternal grandmother made a suicide attempt and was hospitalised. After her death, empty brandy bottles were found littered throughout her house.

My father endured depression and alcoholism, while my uncle suffers from agoraphobia and obsessive-compulsive disorder.

I conclude, then, that there is a genetic inheritance within my family that predisposes its recipients to emotional disturbance. But what form does this legacy take? It could be understood as a direct legacy of the depressive gene TH5. However, psychologist Elaine Aron[14] has persuaded me to appreciate it as an inherited tendency towards high sensitivity shared by about 20 per cent of the population. This characteristic derives from a central nervous system predisposed to elevated responses towards environmental stimulus, and which is associated with artistic and creative temperaments.

Now, genetic seeds grow differently according to the nutrients supplied by an individual's environment. Some highly sensitive people's lives enable them to develop their creative talents. But children whose family circumstances are stressful are more likely to suffer trauma that gives rise to depression. Trauma is a relative term referring to how an event is interpreted rather than to some objective measure.

My father's vulnerable temperament manifested as depression/alcoholism after a claustrophobic childhood and nightmarish wartime experiences. In my case, a genetic predisposition towards sensitivity was transformed into anxiety/depression by the shock of a life-saving operation at the age of three weeks and by insecure attachment with my somewhat depressed mother. This laid the foundations for a learnt self-critical and pessimistic life script. As I grew older, I experienced the emotional chaos of a family with an alcoholic father, which is associated with depressive inclinations in children.

At the age of three weeks, I started to projectile vomit and lost weight rapidly being unable to retain food. My mother describes me as being literally only skin and bones. I was suffering from pyloric stenosis, a condition that required immediate surgery. Subsequently, the anaesthetic caused severe congestion of the lungs; I coughed endlessly and my parents took it in turns to sit with me every night for two years. My mother tells me she was terrified the day I was taken into hospital. She remained anxious during the period of my recovery and reports that the next two years were a period of sleep deprivation and marital tension. Despite this, she breastfed me every two hours for the first nine months of my life.

None can be sure about the effects of these events on my life, but there is evidence that an operation in the early days of life can have lifelong psychobiological consequences. Attachment research has found that negative life events are an important factor in establishing insecure attachment styles. Among such events are: a life-threatening illness for the child, the inconsistent emotional availability of parents and a parental psychiatric disorder.

My father was an alcoholic and I felt that he wielded arbitrary power over me in an unjust manner. Whether fairly or not, I experienced him as disapproving, controlling and just a bit scary. By my teenage years, he was telling me what to do and I was resisting. My mother is strong, competent and very loyal in some ways, yet deeply insecure in others. She does not show joy or pleasure easily in her face, which often appears as worried, withdrawn and depressed. Faces are important signals for an infant and allow them to become attached to their mothers. It is likely that as a sick child I found it hard to connect emotionally to my troubled and apprehensive mother. Certainly, my experience of depression is consistent with an anxious/ambivalent attachment style.

My purpose here is to put forward a likely *causal* explanation and not to attach any kind of blame. I am also suggesting that depression originates in more subtle and prosaic ways than overt family trauma. My childhood was not as dangerous as Ben's, and nor were those of executives to whom I spoke, yet some of them had also experienced depression.

Successful men also get depressed

Twenty-five per cent of the executives told me that they had suffered from depression at some point in their lives. This is just above the national average and considerably exceeds the reported figures for men (but has no statistical validity). Four of five executives who described bouts of anxiety/depression indicated predispositions (genetic inheritance and family psychology) that were evident in childhood. Nonetheless, tendencies require environmental triggers, which include the stress and relative isolation of their lives.

Tony (aged 48, a chief executive officer) told me: 'Sometimes I'd just burst into tears, driving home in the car, I'd just burst into tears and I obviously wasn't coping. There is no doubt in my mind now. But at the same time I wasn't a disaster.' Tony's company provided a counselling service for its employees, but he was reluctant to talk to them. Depression remains a condition that we are not inclined to draw to our employers' attention — often with good reason. However, Tony recognised that he was depressed and eventually sought assistance. He changed career for a couple of years, entering a less stressed environment before returning to the executive fold.

Tony learnt to take regular exercise and to attend to his self-talk as ways of combating depression. That is, he learnt to pay attention to the stream of thoughts that flowed through his mind in order to be able to step back and consider their validity. This is an important skill for depression sufferers, since it is our own self-critical thoughts of inadequacy that bring us down. Tony also recognised that, behind the self-confident front of his colleagues, 'a lot of people don't actually know any more or are any more capable, regardless of what they say and the way they posture, you know, get behind the bullshit and everyone has kind of fears and doubts'. So Tony was able to put his own anxieties into a proper perspective.

Brian (aged 35, a senior accountant) told me of an 18-month period when he was very depressed, had no friends and never went out socially. 'I had a very low opinion of my capabilities and I think I was depressed over a long period of time,' he said. However, the depression eventually lifted, not least because the higher education training he had been undertaking resulted in good grades, a boost in self-confidence and a new job. But depression is prone to recurrence and Brian told me that he was again feeling stressed, agitated and angry to the point where his girlfriend was expressing her concern. And a shortage of time in his busy work-oriented life meant he had stopped the jogging that had previously combated stress. Brian's anxiety and depression owed a good deal to the fact that his sense of self-worth was tied to successful public performance.

PERFORMANCE ANXIETY

We now locate 'success' and 'failure' in the psychology and moral worth of individuals rather than in an externally determined 'Fate'. Indeed, the institutions of our society compel us to develop a personal biography. We are addressed as individual consumers who must make wise choices; we are expected to manage individual careers; and traditional relationship bonds have given way to personalised negotiations.

This process of 'individuation' promises freedom of choice and the creative construction of a life path through developing personal talents. However, it also brings the pressures of decision-making in a world where certainties (for example, of church, family and moral codes) have collapsed. Without reliable foundations for our choices, how do we know which ones to make? What is our value if we are ordinary and not extraordinary? This is the 'age of anxiety' – and anxiety is the flip side of depression.

The rise of individualism is a key factor accounting for increased depression in the Western world, where we measure worth through money, public visibility and winning. Personal achievement is highly valued and deemed to be a consequence of individual effort. We are a part of a heroic culture in which accomplishments are attributed to 'special' people who deserve their rewards. These notions of personal triumph underpin widespread anxiety about self-worth: any performance that falls short of self-expectations can easily be interpreted as personal 'failure'.

William: Running from 'failure'

In chapter 2, I suggested that relatively low levels of depression found among sportsmen reflected purposeful outward-looking attitudes, participation in a social network of like-minded people and the antidepressant qualities of physical activity. We noted that there is scientific evidence and personal testimony that exercise makes us feel better. And we met William, a 30-year-old athlete who described how running made him 'feel heaps better' and how he loved 'the peak feeling that it gives you'. However, while one may set goals and drive oneself forwards, not everyone succeeds. There is a thin line between 'thinking positively' in order to get the best out of life and making unrealistic demands on oneself. How does one then cope with a sense of 'failure'?

William joined his local athletics club at the age of 13, beginning a routine of regular training and competition that lasted for many years. He was particularly adept at running 400 and 800 metre races, winning at local and state levels. William's social world was organised around athletics and his achievements radically boosted his self-esteem. At university, under the guidance of his coach, he won a national title and set his sights on the Olympic team. However, a nagging groin injury worsened and ruled him out of athletics, and with it his Olympic hopes.

> I had in mind that I could make the Olympic team, but the injury was too bad. I couldn't run, it was detrimental, so I just gave it away at one stage. It was a big disappointment, yeah, because I had the dream of making the Olympics and the possibility was there but I couldn't do it because of an injury. (William, aged 30)

The disappointment of missing out on Olympic participation was so great that William turned his back on athletics entirely: 'I went overseas for six months to do something completely different with my life.' He considered that six months abroad as one of the best times of his life because it completely removed any pressure to succeed. On his return, the injury had still not recovered sufficiently for him to be able to compete at an international level. 'I was depressed and upset about it; it was a life dream of mine and I wasn't able to achieve it,' he said. Indeed, it took five years and the assistance of a therapist before he returned to athletics.

PESSIMISM AND OPTIMISM

Whether one considers winning national championships but just missing out on the Olympic team as a 'successful' athletics career or as a 'failure' depends on one's point of view. As psychologist Martin Seligman[15] (see chapter 5) explains, an optimist regards difficulties as specific to particular circumstances and beyond their control. They will say: 'I had a great time and I was unlucky that my talent was restricted by injury. I'll have better luck with my new venture.' Pessimists think that problems are a pervasive and permanent feature of their lives caused by their own actions. A pessimist will say: 'Of course I failed to make the Olympic team. Things always go wrong for me because I am so stupid. I should never have done so much training.'

Learnt pessimism is strongly associated with depression. It stems from the helplessness a child feels when they sense that whatever they do will not attract the love and care they need. It is no surprise, then, to learn that the young men from the drop-in centre saw life's glass as half empty. Nonetheless, even pessimists can learn to maintain emotional wellbeing by periodically renegotiating their life goals. Since only a very few of us reach the highest peaks of 'success', we must learn to distance ourselves from too rigid an interpretation of achievement and failure.

We come to accept that disappointment is an inevitable fact of life, and then redefine success. To do so, we need to sidestep our 'achievement culture' and its associated anxiety by developing alternative values and visions of accomplishment. For example, if we don't achieve that much sought-after promotion, we may decide that our family life is more important to us, or we may find renewed pleasure in gardening or painting. William was eventually able to redefine his yardstick for success and failure. After his Olympic disappointments, he trained as a teacher, developing new goals and gratifications guiding young athletes.

> My whole aim was to make the Olympics when I was younger and I think that was a goal set too high. Now I know that I just have to set little achievements and goals and I am happy with whatever I can do now. (William, aged 30)

Tom had ambitions to play hockey at an international level and, although he played for the state side, the national team eluded him. Tom was disappointed, but unlike William, he did not become depressed. Instead, he made a decision to give more time to study and downgraded his sporting ambitions.

> At heart, I knew it was a touch-and-go thing, but I also made a conscious decision about whether to go full-on for hockey or to study. I made

a conscious decision to study, not to abandon hockey but to put it in perspective. I have a sense of always trying to balance my life and I guess the decision I was faced with then could have tipped it out of balance. (Tom, aged 38)

Tom adopted a less destructive way to cope with setbacks than did William. The young men at the drop-in centre and the older men from the rest home had similarly differential responses to trauma.

Trauma and resilience

The suicide rate among men has two peaks: first with young men aged between 20 and 25 and again among men over 80 years of age. Elderly men face an inevitable sense of loss with the demise of loved ones and the prospect of their own imminent death. Yet, strangely enough, depression was mentioned only twice in my conversations with Diggers. This relatively low incidence of talk about despair was in distinct contrast to the 20-year-olds from the drop-in centre. I wondered why this was so, especially as the lives of the elderly men were marked by traumatic experiences.

A CONVENIENT FORGETTING

Throughout human history, war has been a central component of male experience, leaving its mark through what we now call 'post-traumatic stress disorder'. Certainly, war was a defining moment for this Digger generation, and for my father whose own experiences in the British Army contributed to his alcoholism.

Harold (aged 75) told me that the war was a 'low-key affair' for him: 'If you are thinking I have any traumatic … well, no. That's all I can say.' Yet, perhaps this is just forbearance, since 'when I was demobbed I wanted to forget it, to put it completely and thoroughly behind me. I wouldn't even join the RSL [Retired Servicemen's League]'. Though war is hardly a routine experience, Harold claimed to have 'put it out of my mind'. Nonetheless, about one in five men are seriously traumatised by war, and these are likely to be the men described by Aron as highly sensitive.

'I had no fear of war,' declared 77-year-old Eddy. 'It was just a job. You fight for your country.' Yet, I wonder if Eddy wasn't simply evading his troubles, since he was an alcoholic, a condition probably exasperated by his wartime experience. The men from the Diggers Rest Home were generally talkative and open about their lives, but persuading them to talk about war was more challenging. 'It's not a thing I like speaking a lot about,' said Max (aged 87). 'Most of the men that served on the Kokoda Trail that I rubbed shoulders with were very quiet, they wouldn't speak.' Max had spent time in a Japanese POW camp, but claimed that 'I can't remember too much about prison life' and 'I didn't have any traumatic experiences'. Of course, this may be true. However, given what we now know about trauma, it is more plausible to understand this as a 'convenient' forgetting. Yet, there was also a streak of stoicism and resilience among some of these men that enabled them to survive the horror.

EDWARD: WITH ACCEPTANCE AND RESISTANCE

Edward fought in the army against the Japanese during the Second World War and until he was captured. He was imprisoned and used as forced labour building railways along with thousands of other POWs, many of whom perished amid atrocious conditions.

> We don't talk a lot about our experiences up in the islands. I thought when I came here, I thought the old buggers would talk about their experiences up in the islands; what they did and what they didn't do. But you don't want to remember a lot of it; they were bad times. The one alongside of you got knocked down and you were still standing there and I couldn't understand it; it's a strange thing. (Edward, aged 89)

However, as Edward explained: 'You put it behind you, you have to. If you don't, you've had it. We had to face up to most things and we had to take them in our stride.' 'We had to wear them as they came,' he said. 'It's surprising what you can take if you have to.' Yet, it was many years before Edward was able to remember or talk about his experiences.

> I couldn't talk about it like I can now. I had all the memories and I couldn't dwell on them until such time as I could sit down and think

about them. When that happened, I was still very much in possession of my memories but I had lost a lot and they were starting to disappear. It was 1975 before I could settle down and write about it. I had stirring memories of it. But something cleared away in the late seventies and I could sit down and write a book. (Edward, aged 89)

Particular personal qualities enabled some men to survive war in emotionally better shape than others. These characteristics include faith, acceptance, will, humour and friendship. For example, in chapter 5 Edward talked about his 'personal relationship with our Lord' that 'strengthened my resolve' and enabled him to survive the Burma Railway and a Japanese POW camp. His Christian faith provided a moral view of the universe and a sense of hope necessary for the buoyancy of spirit required to endure his ordeals with both 'acceptance and resistance'.

JOSHUA: A SPIRITED RESILIENCE

In contrast to Edward, Joshua's (aged 75) three years as a prisoner of the Japanese 'got rid of, definitely, forever and ever, of religion, in the camps. By this I mean organised religion.' Yet, Joshua was one of the most resilient men I have ever met. He was very funny and self-reliant, with 'fuck 'em' as his motto. His resilience derived in part, he suggested, from the fact that 'I was lucky enough to have the cheek to say "Fuck you"'. He described this as a kind of arrogance. 'To this day, I know what arrogance is. Arrogance is a survival technique.' He had developed this attitude as a child in response to his authoritarian father and to a rule-bound boarding school where 'the resistance was enormous. We were resisting; we were rebellious little bastards'. This included publicly urinating in the dining hall and staging a hunger strike. With his father, he 'resisted with Gandhi in my head and a tiger in my bloody heart' in order to break 'the barbed wire of authority'.

Joshua learnt about Gandhi and the spiritual teacher Krishnamurti at the feet of his mother: 'The thing was, I liked Gandhi. I liked what she said about Gandhi and I also felt her incredible admiration for him.' These teachings supported his strong sense of self and the belief that 'each individual has their own channel and that's inside; you should listen to this person and find that channel'. Joshua had a keen sense of survival. This was not rooted in organised religion, and especially not in Christianity, which he distrusted, but was situated in a 'spirituality' mediated through Gandhi, and through his artistic commitments as a painter.

I was struck by Joshua's humour and irreverence for any kind of authority. 'Really, you need two things,' he said, to survive the camps and life: 'you need to keep your bloody head, don't panic and have a sense of humour'. Like Edward, Joshua too was 'spirited'. If we regard spirituality as a set of practices that mould and change the self rather than as unsubstantiated 'belief' systems, then we can understand how it provides practical-moral resources for personal growth and hardiness (see chapter 10). Indeed, hope and a sense of ethical order are essential to the resilience of POW camp survivors.

FACING UP TO LOSS

The elderly men from the rest home had seen their fair share of suffering. They had toiled long hours in demanding jobs (see chapter 8) and seen friends killed in war. Now they were witnessing the death of loved ones, particularly spouses, but even children. Alan lived a happy married life with a woman he loved who constituted the centre of his world. At the age of 45, she was diagnosed with cancer. 'I couldn't believe it,' he said. His wife was being treated in hospital when one day 'they phoned me to tell me to come in as she was pretty low'. He sat with her all that Friday night and into the next day before making a brief visit to the shops because his sisters-in-law were visiting, and he didn't have any food in the house. 'I had just got the shopping done and got back when the phone rang'. It was the ward:

> Your wife has just passed away, they said. I said, 'I'll be in'. My daughter and her husband were already in there. I went in and sobbed, cried. I stayed there for about an hour and a half and they came and dragged me out and that was the last time I saw my Joan. It was sad. (Alan, aged 79)

When Harold's wife Betty died, 'it was a shock, it was a terrible shock. I suppose that I grieved for her much longer than any other person in my life'. These are painful moments, yet somehow people survive them. Harold mourned Betty, but 'I didn't go into decline and within a few months it had passed'. Strangely, it was the death of his cat that provoked his greatest sense of loss.

> It's funny, but the thing that brought me so much grief, when I think of the death of people that I love, was this: a pussycat which I became very fond of. Finally, the cat got sick with kidney disease and nothing could be done. I grieved over that for ages. It's ridiculous, isn't it, that humans can do this. (Harold, aged 75)

As elderly men with physical ailments to remind them of their fragility, the Diggers now face their own mortality. Confronting death involves a series of emotional strategies that include anger, denial, negotiation, depression and acceptance. These feelings do not necessarily appear consecutively, but cycle around each other. For example, Edward said with acceptance 'I am just waiting for the end', but with the very next breath he was talking about writing another book. Harold didn't want to die and was 'not looking forward to it', but nonetheless was able to say that 'I don't feel frightened by it'. Death was a reality that was simultaneously accepted and denied. As Charlie (aged 88) said, 'I don't know if I accept it or not. It's not on your mind, even though you see it all the time.'

Depression in changing times

The Diggers were a generation of men that suffered hardship and from whose ranks we might have expected to hear more stories of depression. Yet, for many of them stoicism, acceptance and emotional discipline enabled resilience more than despair. Nevertheless, a number of the Diggers did respond to emotional pain with addictions such as drinking and gambling. While these elderly men did not speak much about depression, they did talk a lot about widespread alcohol misuse (see chapter 7). Many of the older men who developed alcohol dependency were using it, like my father, to mask depression and/or post-traumatic stress disorder.

Similarly, the drug users from the drop-in centre were using heroin to deal with depression, and yet they were more able to recognise this process than were the Diggers. This may be a facet of different patterns of drug use; perhaps alcohol masks depression more than does heroin. But I would suggest that it is better explained as a generational cultural phenomenon. That is, younger men are more willing to talk about depression than are older men.

Despite the stigma that continues to surround it, we are able to talk about depression today more readily than when the Diggers were in their formative years. The psychological language of depression and parenting/childhood has seeped into popular culture via magazines such as *Cosmopolitan* or *Men's Health* and television shows like *Oprah*, *Dr Phil* and *Jerry Springer*. Even soap operas like *Neighbours* and *The Bold and the Beautiful* or dramas such as *The OC* feature the new cultural language of self-help psychology. The young men at the drop-in centre had a familiarity with 'psychology talk' and felt more comfortable with it than their elderly counterparts. Indeed, they may even be recycling a psychological 'script' as an explanation for their own behaviour.

DEPRESSION YOUNG AND OLD

Nevertheless, the higher rate of depression talk among the younger men does, I think, reflect genuinely higher incidences of depression; a significant reason for which is found in their respective backgrounds. All the young heroin users had unhealthy patterns of parenting and disturbed childhoods, whereas this was the case for only a minority of the Diggers. This directs our attention once again to the foundational character of family life for emotional health. Men whose adult lives were apparently more traumatic than those of the drug users were better psychologically equipped to survive because of their established emotional solidity. It is not simply our 'objective' experience that counts, but our attitudes towards it. It is pertinent, then, to consider a contrast in mindsets between the two groups of men.

The young men and the Diggers both hailed from relatively poor working-class environments. However, the latter were more stoical in the face of hardship; they expected less. Today, we live in a culture that has increased 'choices' in life. We now have more material goods on offer and higher expectations of personal achievement. We compare our lifestyle more with others and expect to have as much as, if not more than, our neighbours. In short, I am suggesting that the lower expectations and greater acceptance of elderly men provided them with a degree of psychological immunisation against depression. Or, to put the proposition the other way round: a culture that contains greater expectations of personal success and less acceptance of hardship will experience more psychological distress. This is particularly so for young men whose relative economic and cultural 'failure' was visible to them.

The Diggers entered into the workforce at a young age by today's standards. They were occupied and subject to the discipline of older men. And however hard it was working on the railways or down the mines, it was at least felt to be purposeful. These men felt useful. Similarly, wartime military service is unwelcome and can be severely traumatic, but many of the Diggers did feel that it was necessary and meaningful to them. The higher incidence of Christian faith among the Diggers also provided some of them with a commitment lacking in the younger men. A sense of purpose is central to a happy life (see chapter 10) and the young men from the drop-in centre had not experienced their social worth in the company of adult men. Nor had they been required or been able to develop much self-discipline.

The quality of love

Depression among men is an increasingly visible feature of contemporary life. Genetic disposition plays a part in this malaise. However, this is an insufficient explanation for the growth of depression in Western cultures. The way we think is the more powerful cause of depression, which in turn has its roots in our childhood families. And there is something not quite right about many families in our society.

I am not suggesting that any particular family form is the only one that works. I am not arguing for a return to conservative family values. Indeed, the 'conventional' family has been the crucible of violence, emotional deprivation and depression. Rather, I am pointing to the *quality of love* in all relationships as being critical to the wellbeing of individuals and cultures. Love requires an intention to forge human connection through understanding, care and attention; but it also implies that we have the skills to turn intention into actuality. We need to learn how to love. The dark night of depression can lead men into self-destruction. However, it can also prompt a period of self-reflection, readjustment and the acquisition of more skilful means of emotional management. In particular, a loving form of 'spirituality' can emerge from an encounter with despair, as we shall see in chapter 11.

Emotional strategies that develop within families are mediated through the cultural configurations of particular times and places. In particular, our current emphasis on individualism and material wealth in the context of growing uncertainty is amplifying 'affective disorders'. Individuation may increase the opportunities for self-fashioning, but it also cuts us off from each other. Because of their external orientation and attachment to ideas of achievement, performance and work, men are particularly prone to social isolation. And this forms one of the conditions for alcohol and drug dependency, the theme of our next chapter.

Living on drugs and alcohol

'Every crime I committed has been under the influence of alcohol. I know it's my biggest downfall,' said 31-year-old Toby, an Indigenous Australian adopted by a white Christian family at the age of two weeks.

> At the age of 14, I left home because that's when I started rebelling and I was starting to get into alcohol and I started hanging around the wrong group at school. That's when I first got into crime, hanging around the group: that was a break and enter and I got charged for it. (Toby, aged 31)

Toby first went into jail when he was 18, returning intermittently over the next four years, at which point he tried to settle down with his partner:

> I had a beautiful girlfriend and I was keeping out of trouble, doing the right thing, trying to make a go of life. When she broke up with me, I took to the grog again, 'cause I felt broken-hearted, shattered, 'cause I was really in love with this woman. I had no money on me, so I ended up stealing a car going back to Sydney and on the way to Sydney I got pulled over and I got charged for car stealing. (Toby, aged 31)

And so it was back to jail for Toby, a pattern he was to repeat over the next eight years. On one of the occasions when he was not in prison, he was convicted of assaulting a police officer.

> This copper tried to tackle me and I pulled the knife out and stabbed him in the arm and then I held him hostage for five hours. When I went to court, the judge said to me, 'Why did you stab the policeman?' and I said, 'Because I wanted to do it and I was under the influence of alcohol'. I had to take all these drugs to calm me down, because I had to see a psychiatrist and they put it down as 'post-traumatic stress disorder' and I had flashbacks from my childhood. My childhood was hard and strict. I was always flogged and I've seen sexual assault happen in my house with my twin sister. That's what screwed my head up.
>
> I got out in December this year and I've been doing well. I don't drink. I'll probably have one stubby a day, if that. It has scared me. I haven't got the taste for it anymore, it don't interest me. This time around, well, you know how I was adopted out, next week I'm heading up there to meet my family for the first time. I'm looking forward to it. After 30 years not knowing who I am, I realise now my identity. If I don't do this, my spirit won't rest. (Toby, aged 31)

We are all drug users. Few people in our culture have not used tea, coffee, alcohol, antibiotics and paracetamol, for example. Even the use of an illegal drug such as marijuana is now widespread. Though former US President Clinton may not have inhaled, he did admit to smoking cannabis. Meanwhile, the pharmaceutical industry sells us tablets to ease the symptoms of stress in the age of Prozac (an antidepressant) and Ritalin (for attention deficit hyperactivity disorder). The central issue is not whether we use drugs per se; after all, where would modern medicine be without them? The crucial question is what place drugs have in our lives. What singles out Toby and the young heroin addicts is not so much that they are drug users, but rather social condemnation, the severity of the narcotic effects and the organising place of drug use in their lives. In so far as drug use is detrimental to their physical and mental health, it is reasonable to move from the word 'use' to 'abuse'. In that sense, *all* the young men from the drop-in centre were current or former drug abusers, with alcohol, marijuana, amphetamine and heroin being the main drugs of choice, often in combination.

John's descent into hell

John's mother had been married 'four or five times' and there were between five and six kids in the house at any one time. John had brothers and sisters who he had never met. His most recent stepfather was an ex-Vietnam veteran suffering from post-traumatic stress disorder, which manifested itself through alcohol abuse and violence. Although John told me that he had a good relationship with his mother, he had repeatedly run away from home. This set the stage for a series of family confrontations.

> I would come home drunk or stoned. I was running amuck. Making a mess and hurling abuse if she wanted me to do something. I was a proper little shit. I just didn't understand it at the time and I was pretty much drugged at that stage when I got kicked out. (John, aged 21)

Drug use began early in life for these young men, sometimes while they were at primary school and certainly by the start of their teens. In school, John described himself as 'the class clown, I was interested in making people laugh instead of doing my work'. He was in continual trouble and frequently ran away.

> I was kicked out at 13 and just started doing what I wanted to do. Actually, about a year before that I was pissed off because I had a fight with the old lady and I ended up moving in with my brother, 'cause I was on the streets for a while, just hanging around. A man took me to some foster place and I stayed there for one night and got out the window the next day and pissed off. I stayed with my brother for a while and afterwards I moved out for good, about a year later and I haven't been back since. (John, aged 21)

John told me that he was 'always stoned from a young age'. By the time he was 13, he was smoking marijuana daily. At 14, he was a heroin addict and remained so when he was 21. From the age of 13, John had no stable home: he travelled around and lived on the streets or in the houses of friends. He had found it difficult to remain in even municipal housing because the public money he received was insufficient to meet his growing drug habits, let alone pay the rent. Consequently, he funded his addiction through burglary, shoplifting and prostitution. He was known to the police and had a few minor convictions, but had spent only two months in detention. However, his lifestyle was taking its toll:

> I think I'm gonna die, I don't know. I've got some sickness. I'm pretty sure I've got Hepatitis C. It has really affected me already, like it's painful, you know, sometimes, mostly in the morning, I'm not sure. I don't see a future anymore; I used to see one. I'm 21 and I feel very old, I feel like I'm deteriorating already, like I'm old, which is not right. Most of the time I just sit there thinking 'When is the day gonna end?' and then some days I think 'Shit, if I do this all the time I really am gonna be old' and think 'What happened?'. I've done a lot of stupid things, a lot of shit. It's just so bad that lifestyle. You do need a break from it and I haven't had a break from that lifestyle for years now. (John, aged 21)

Despite the realisation that he was damaging himself, John was unable to relinquish his heroin habit. He was caught in a vicious cycle of emotional suffering. Without hope, he could not see himself becoming 'clean', but without being clean he had no prospects of the job, house and steady relationship that he thought would be the basis for a heroin-free existence. He could imagine a life without being high:

> Only if I had some sort of job to boost my spirit, just to make me happy, because I don't have any plans, no goals, nothing. I just hope I don't have HIV or something like that, I really do. I do feel like I'm dying, I feel like I'm sick. (John, aged 21)

'I know I like to get stoned, I always have,' he told me. 'I am not really sure why.' Yet, 'heaps of nightmares' during childhood in which 'I was shit scared but I don't know why' offer a clue to the origins of his addictions. He lived in a chaotic family of many children and three different fathers in which the stepfather 'gave out beltings'. A feature of these unhappy families mentioned by 20 per cent of the young men was the occurrence of sexual abuse. They did not venture much by way of details, and I did not think it appropriate to press them, but the consequences in terms of anger, depression and drug abuse were as predictable as the coming of dawn.

> It was me real father but I hadn't said nothing 'cause I was too young to even know what it was, but once I started getting a bit older and I knew it was wrong and then it just got too much and I just blurted it out to my mum one day and she just said, 'I don't believe you' and I just looked at her and said, 'You're kidding, Mum, do you think I make up stories like this every day?' and she said, 'No, but I still don't believe you' and I just walked out and I didn't go home for about five months. It's degrading, it's like someone has taken advantage of you in the most vulnerable situation as being a child who can't defend themselves and when you do get the courage and they don't believe you, well, that shatters your dignity and everything. It makes you not want to live no more and most people like me have already tried and some succeed and some don't and I didn't, but I'm glad I didn't. (John, aged 21)

PHILIP: YOU DON'T HAVE TO WORRY ABOUT ANYTHING NO MORE

John's story of family trauma was not an isolated instance among the young drug users, but rather a paradigm case. For example, Philip (aged 24) was kicked out of home at the age of 14 and had been living on the streets. In his family, he 'got blamed for everything and I got hit a lot'. Family conflict fuelled by drug and alcohol abuse was a common feature of these young men's lives. Philip's father was an alcoholic (see chapter 4) and the politics of the family eventually led to his being homeless.

> I started arguing with my dad. I hated him and he hated me. We used to have punch-ups and stuff. My dad would come and complain about me and smash me around. He was always the sort of person that if I didn't do anything to his standards, like if I wasn't good enough, he'd go mad. He used to drink and smoke pot and stuff like that. I don't know, he just started being a real bastard to me and I started arguing with him and the more I argued with him the more Mum would get it. My mum said one day, like she practically chose, she had to choose between me and him. She chose him in the end, 'cause she reckons that it was all my fault that their relationship was splitting up and everything. So they just about told me to leave. (Philip, aged 24)

'Compared to there, the streets are virtually luxury, 'cause you don't get beaten around and it's not like the house is all messy,' he said. Nevertheless, his sense of loss remained: 'I see some families and I get jealous.' He had his first experience of marijuana three days after he left home and continued because 'it would help me sleep at night'. He was then introduced to speed (amphetamine) and heroin. The appeal of heroin was that 'it numbs you so you don't have to worry about anything no more'.

Addiction as defence

Men learn to seek self-esteem through public recognition. The relentless critical self-monitoring this demands, whether that be at work or in bed, manifests as grandiosity on the one hand and deep feelings of inadequacy on the other (for the performances are never outstanding enough to satisfy the internal parents). The flip side of the culture of achievement is the need to take flight from the pressures of constant self-appraisal through compulsive behaviours (addictions) centred on work and drugs.

Addiction and other forms of compulsive behaviour offer a source of comfort and a defence against anxiety, so that failure to engage in them produces an upsurge of dread and/or depression. The workaholism of 'successful' executives and the drug abuse of social 'failures' are two sides of the same coin. As British sociologist Anthony Giddens explains[1], addictions are narcotic-like time-outs that blunt the pain of longings that cannot be directly controlled. For example, Toby and John use drugs to disassociate themselves from the emotional suffering of childhood sexual abuse. And below we meet executives who use alcohol to escape the stress of continued decision-making.

Addiction is an escape from the responsibility for continual choice that accompanies the development of an autonomous self. The addictive experience is a search for that 'high' that enables us to 'give up' the self and be released from its anxieties. It marks a temporary abandonment of the continued self-monitoring that is entrenched in contemporary life. For Giddens, 'Every addiction is a defensive reaction, and an escape, a recognition of lack of autonomy that casts a shadow over the competence of the self'.[2] This suspension of the self is frequently followed by feelings of shame and remorse. Since addiction signals incapacity to cope with anxieties, they tend to be functionally interchangeable; one overthrows an addiction only to replace it with another.

ADDICTED TO WORDS

The distinctions between John, my father and myself are simply matters of degree. We occupy slightly different positions on a drug-using continuum, but we do not inhabit completely alien worlds. I have adopted a number of defensive strategies against my own anxiety. One has been the development of an intellectualism that at its root seeks to control the world and restrict its fearful unpredictability. Ever since I was a child, I have enjoyed the illuminating force of language. I have used words as both sword and shield. My father, who preferred a good whisky to a good read, sneered at my preference for books over machinery. Worse, he feared words, seeing in their dexterous use some hidden accusation; he retaliated with sticks and stones.

But words are unruly and disorderly creatures. They take on a life of their own, picking up momentum until with growing velocity they fill the mind with an infinite stream of nightmare visions and grandiose scenarios. Thus does the web that was spun to keep the world at bay turn on its creator like lantana of the mind: a thicket that cuts out the light of the world and strangles the spirit. With words we may conjure up great beauty and lighten the heart, but we may also bring forth the darkness and deepen the fear. Words need to be disciplined and used with care. Words need to be forged on the anvil of poetry.

My wordy strategy has the benefit of social commendation and external validation, allowing me to be a 'good boy'. Another 'defence', if it can be called such, has been to sink into a depression that, painful though it is, has put a temporary end to anxiety. This has, of course, taken me out of the frying pan and into the fire. And if not books or depression, then drugs and alcohol as self-medication; I have had periods in my life when I have abused both alcohol and marijuana.

Good boy turned bad – after all, I also had a rebellious streak. As a teenager, I was 'rebel boy' and drove my father mad by growing my hair long and adopting the radical politics of the late 1960s. In fact, I was generally resistant to all male authority figures. Finally, along with other men, I have sought to ameliorate anxiety and fill the void of loneliness through sex. In any case, all these compulsive strategies seek solutions from without – and this is their major failing (see chapters 10 and 11).

The sociability of drugs

In our culture, alcohol is intrinsic to most social occasions. We meet friends at the pub or in a restaurant for dinner and a glass of wine. Alcohol is woven into the very fabric of social life, whereby we signal approval of drug use as a social lubricant. The illegal drug scene is also a social experience and not simply a source of intoxication. The young men I talked with knew each other as part of a community that offered friendship and support.

> I liked the feeling and it put me in the same category as other people. I could walk down the street and see someone else and have a good yarn. So it all ended up in one big circle and started with mates and ended with mates: the circle got bigger, at least my circle did. (David, aged 29)

Of course, this social network also makes drugs available and generates a mutual encouragement to use. The recurrent advice offered by men who have successfully relinquished illegal drug use – and many of these men had done so periodically – is to leave the neighbourhood and get out of the 'scene'. But it is hard enough to free oneself of addiction at the best of times, but even tougher to do so without established friends. The role of drugs in a social network is just as strong, of course, among corporate executives as it is among young heroin users. For businessmen, alcohol is a social lubricant providing a medium for friendship and a defence against loneliness.

JAMES: I GAMBLE A BIT UNDER PRESSURE

James (aged 49, chief financial officer of a major Australian company) told me that he didn't have any real friends at work: 'I mix with lots of people, and I've got colleagues right across the world, but I don't have anyone close here.

> I think one of the mistakes you make in business is that you keep up this pace and oomph, you try stopping and then you find that you haven't spent enough time developing your friendships, developing your relationships. I have a narrow group of friends; I don't have time to develop new friends, I just don't. (James, aged 49)

James described himself as a heavy drinker at the age of 16, to the extent that his father had to 'pick me up off the front porch and carry me inside'. By the time he married at 22, this intense phase had passed, though he did still drink alcohol daily. He observed that booze still troubled his brother, suggesting a family predisposition towards dependency. James also told me about high levels of anxiety and panic attacks he had experienced, though he attributed this to his deteriorating marriage rather than to the pressures of work. Nevertheless, there is a suggestion here of a 'hard-wired' tendency towards anxiety met by addiction.

> I gamble a bit when under pressure and I can develop a bit of a gambling problem. Sometimes I have a problem with my gambling, like when I was commuting down to Melbourne I started gambling too much because you work a long day, you walk back to the motel room, sit around, so you go down to the Casino or something like that. So, yeah, that's happened now and again, but I just need to bring it under control. (James, aged 49)

FRANK'S NORMAL DRINKING

A striking feature of these executives' lives was the absence of a developed friendship network. Indeed, a number of them told me that they had agreed to our discussion because it provided an anonymous space in which to talk. This is not to say that they had no social life, since corporate functions filled their diaries. However, business gatherings are not usually spaces for personal intimacy and carry the temptations of alcohol abuse.

All the executives agreed heavy workloads, long hours, pressuring deadlines and high performance expectations constituted high-stress lives. In this context, a lack of social support and low levels of physical activity (only two men did regular exercise) is a recipe for alcohol abuse and/or depression. Two of the men said that they used marijuana and a couple of others hinted that they did but would not elaborate. However, all of the executives said that alcohol was a regular part of their lives. Most felt that their drinking was normal, reasonable and not out of control despite its daily practice. As Frank explained:

> I probably should develop some outside interests. I don't do enough sport and that kind of thing. I do know how to go out and have a good evening, but that's probably not as healthy as punishing a squash ball, not to oblivion but you can take the edge off the situation. Most nights when I get home I'll have a beer or a gin and tonic or something; which if that was all I drank that night would probably be good for me. I drink every day; you know, if I have a gin and tonic or a glass and a half of red wine with dinner, that is probably fine. Probably the textbooks would say that's a unit or two too much, but not a problem; then, of course, you go to a party and lose count. (Frank, aged 43)

Consuming beer or wine every day was the norm for these men. As Maurice (aged 37) put it: 'Alcohol, I'd have a few drinks every day, I guess, and I mean maybe it's the social mantra of Australia, a couple of beers.' Daily drinking could be seen as addiction, because it is regular and compulsive, even though it falls within the norms of the cultural milieu. Since alcohol is an intrinsic part of the business world and of the recreational activities of our culture more generally, we may observe that addiction is a mainstream condition. Two of the men said that they had faced problems with alcohol in the past, but they were sure that it was not alcoholism, and it was no longer an issue – well, not really.

The lonely glass

My father is standing in the doorway swaying gently with the uncertain movements of a newborn calf. Convinced that no one knows where he's been, his deluded mind edges unsteadily forward on disobedient legs. But his faraway glassy eyes and the belligerence of his voice tell me all I need to know. It would be best to be unobtrusive and slip quietly away to my room, but there is the fantasy of a family meal to be endured: a simulacrum of normality, a copy of an original that never existed. I sit at the table hoping that nothing is said or done to crack open the hallucination and let forbidden reality through. May I please not spill my drink or drop my food or in any way incite his anger. May my mother not come to my defence, only to be abused for her trouble. May I contain my fearful anger. May it all be over soon.

When I was a boy, my father's drinking scared me. He looked disturbing, he smelled strange and he would become unpredictable and threatening. My father's alcoholism was not immediately apparent to me as a child. However, by the time I was ten it had emerged into the lounge from the dark corner of his lonesome bedroom in which it had secretly festered. As I grew up, I became progressively angrier with him. Fear and anger are not a good basis for a father–son relationship and from my late teens onwards we hardly spoke. But still, as time has passed and I have looked more deeply at him, myself and my family, I have concluded that today he would be diagnosed as suffering from post-traumatic stress disorder.

Post-traumatic stress disorder is a complex condition whose symptoms include repeated 'flashbacks' or dreams that relive the trauma, and the experience of disassociation or trance-like emotional 'numbness'. It can involve detachment from other people and avoidance of activities and situations reminiscent of the trauma. There can be acute bursts of fear, panic or aggression and there is usually a state of heightened arousal, vigilance and insomnia. Post-traumatic stress disorder is complicated by the fact that it frequently occurs in conjunction with related disorders such as anxiety, depression and substance abuse that also impair a person's ability to function in social and family life.

My father served in the British Army during the Second World War, an experience my mother says he loathed. On the second day of the D-day landings in France, he saw his best friend killed at his shoulder and on returning to civilian life, he suffered from repeated nightmares. My mother says that he would wake up in the middle of the night sweating and shouting out to his mate. I do not recall him having any real friends and he was visibly uncomfortable on social occasions, which he avoided if he could. The older he got, the more time he spent alone in his room drinking. At best, he would fall asleep; at worst, he would emerge from his isolation seeking connection with his family, only to reap the bitter fruits of the havoc he had sowed.

I have little doubt that post-traumatic stress disorder played its part in my father's dislocated life, transforming a genetic predisposition towards sensitivity into alcoholism. The cycle of his suffering has no clear beginning, but my father's anxieties led him into conflict at work and with his wife, which in turn fuelled his depressive drinking. The more isolated he got, the more he sought to drown his fear in alcohol. At least, that is how it now appears to me: a narrative that has the merits of enabling forgiveness and recovering happier memories of football and flickering flames.

For years, I was unable to appreciate that the promise of company took my father to the pub on his way home from work, while drinking at home covered up the demons of his unwelcome solitude in the very place where he felt he should find love and solace, but did not. This is a scenario that fits a number of the Diggers who were of the same generation as my father, had fought in the Second World War and whose relationships with women were caught up in a cycle of loneliness and alcohol abuse.

EDDY AND PUB CULTURE

The pub was the most common place of social interaction for the older generation of men I spoke with. Joe (aged 69) spent a great deal of his life down at the pub drinking and gambling. He had little apparent interest in relationships (he was married once very briefly) and most of the stories that he told concerned alcohol, betting and his mates.

Max described his life as being mainly about work and the pub, which involved 'meeting friends, having company and someone to talk to' (Max, aged 73). In chapter 4, we encountered Eddy, where we learnt about the breakup of his childhood family. Eddy became an alcoholic; but it was not just drink that took him down to the pub, it was also the jovial atmosphere and companionship he found there. This contrasted with a life he described as otherwise 'dull and uninteresting'.

'I lost a lot through grog,' bemoaned Eddy and 'there is a lot of stuff I don't even remember.' Among the things he 'lost' were two wives, a 'de facto' partner and his children (from his first marriage). Music was Eddy's great love, especially the piano, which he played at local pubs in the company of friends. Although he was paid a small fee, the money was secondary to the music and companionship. Eddy had a job as a dental technician and enjoyed his work – until he lost that too. But still, he was having a lot of fun. Unfortunately, his wife was not enjoying life nearly so much, and things became a little fraught at home. However, Eddy was not ready to give up his absentee lifestyle and so, 'I sort of got tied up with another girl' and moved in with her.

Eddy never saw his children again, which remained a source of sadness: 'I missed them. Once you have a few beers, you get a bit morose.' Further, his new relationship was soon over, as 'there was nothing in it, really'. However, music, mates and drinking sustained him until he met Alice, a barmaid, who became his second wife. Now the predictable thing about patterns is that they repeat themselves, and Eddy hopped on the same old roundabout again, throwing in gambling for extra excitement. Even Eddy could see where the marriage was heading: 'Well, I realised that I had messed up the first marriage and the other one was looking like it a lot. She was very good, a lovely person and so I cut back quite a lot.' Indeed, Eddy checked in to a rehab centre to break his addiction and was temporarily successful, but 'the music always won out in the end'.

There was a battle going on inside Eddy between denial and honesty. His explanation that 'he sort of got tied up' with another woman and that it was 'music' rather than alcohol that triumphed looks like self-deception. It wasn't me, he seems to say, it was the malicious forces of unruly fate! On the other hand, the consequences of his actions eventually dawned on him: 'You have to be honest with yourself somewhere along the line. I did the wrong thing. I blame myself. I blame the grog.' Eddy gave up drinking, but not soon enough to save his second marriage; but he did save his liver, just, and thus his life.

It serves no purpose to say that Eddy brought his troubles down on his own head; he is well aware of his shortcomings, and blame does nothing to improve anyone's life. Eddy was not a bad man; no doubt, if he could have behaved differently, he would have. As Iyanla Vanzant writes:

> When you feel sufficiently remorseful, overwhelmingly confused and totally beaten down, you will be on the brink of a divine revelation! You will be face to face with something you probably never considered. The truth is, if you could have done it you would have. The fact that you didn't, means you couldn't, for reasons you may not be aware of right now.[3]

Eddy had painful memories of his parents' separation as a child when 'everything went wrong' (see chapter 4). Further, it was as a soldier that he first started to drink heavily, just like my father.

ALCOHOLISM DESTROYS RELATIONSHIPS

While the Diggers did not talk much about depression, they often used alcohol as a means to ameliorate difficult emotions. Eddy was one of six alcoholics among the 20 (that is, 30 per cent) elderly men that I talked to: a rather high fall-down rate for a small group of men. They had all been married and divorced, with drinking a significant cause of their failed relationships (see chapter 9).

George (aged 74) spent most of his life in the pub drinking and gambling with his mates, and his marriage lasted only six years. Gambling, he said, was more important to him than women. However, this rejection of relationships was a rarity. Ernie (aged 80) had five children and sustained a 28-year marriage, but long periods working away from home, combined with his habitual drinking and gambling, finally led to divorce. Ironically, it was 'having a lot of grog with the father-in-law' that precipitated his downfall. After his wife left him, his drinking got worse and he became estranged from his children. Only two of them, the girls, still talk to him. And yet, Ernie said, his marriage was the most important thing in his life.

Alcohol is often at the centre of our friendship rituals and can oil the wheels of conversation and conviviality. However, it can also destroy relationships. Indeed, for some it played a destructive role within the rest home.

> I won't mention names because it wouldn't be fitting, but there are men here that never give the girls a bit of trouble or the residents, but when they go down and have too much alcohol they come back and they get very aggressive and nasty. I am not a lover of that. (Peter, aged 75)

Peter's distaste for alcohol was embedded in his family history. His father was not a drinker and Peter was raised as a Christian, a stance that he maintained throughout his life. Sadly, Peter witnessed the descent of his uncle Jack, who 'was a wonderful man who never touched alcohol' – until, that is, he returned from First World War military service. Uncle Jack took part in the disastrous Gallipoli landings of April 1915 and survived. Later, he was wounded in France and 'when he came back, you couldn't keep him out of the hotels. I've seen alcohol ruin many a good man' (Peter, aged 75).

Human habits and unwelcome feelings

Human beings seem to like drugs: they may even have had a role in our evolutionary survival. They certainly play a significant part in our cultures. Often drugs are useful to us or can be pleasurably consumed with minimal damage. Yet, drugs can also have severely detrimental consequences. There is no clear line between reasonable drug use and damaging addiction, classifications that can only be social judgments.

Nevertheless, for a significant number of men habitual drug use is such an important, if dangerous, defence against unwelcome feelings that they disrupt their lives and relationships. Many of the problems of male drug abuse, crime and violence in our culture are manifestations of emotional distress. Genetic predispositions play a part in this process.

However, feelings of loss and anxiety rooted in 'insecure attachments' underpin this compulsive behaviour. Family suffering, depression and addiction form a causal circle that plays out a historical game of pass the emotional parcel.

The character of our times shapes the specific ways that emotions are expressed and drugs consumed. For example, the social isolation prevalent in contemporary culture plays a central part in depression and drug use. In particular, the stress of pursuing individualistic careers forms a backdrop to the sustained alcohol consumption of executives. Although alcohol plays a significant part in the male team sports, this particular group of sportsmen showed relatively low levels of alcohol abuse (see chapter 2). Rather, it was among the older generation of men from the rest home that I unearthed a sizeable stream of alcoholism. The younger men from the drop-in centre were more likely to talk about depression than these old soldiers, but their drugs of choice were marijuana and heroin rather than alcohol.

As well as providing the context for our emotional development, culture also offers us explanations for our behaviour. For example, addiction is no longer thought to be the work of evil spirits but of biochemistry and cognitive processes. Today, we look to psychology for a language by which to understand our emotions. Indeed, it is the language of compulsive behaviour drawn from psychology that allows us to see both the consumption of drugs and the compulsion to work as forms of addiction. It is to the latter that we now turn in chapter 8.

Work, work, work

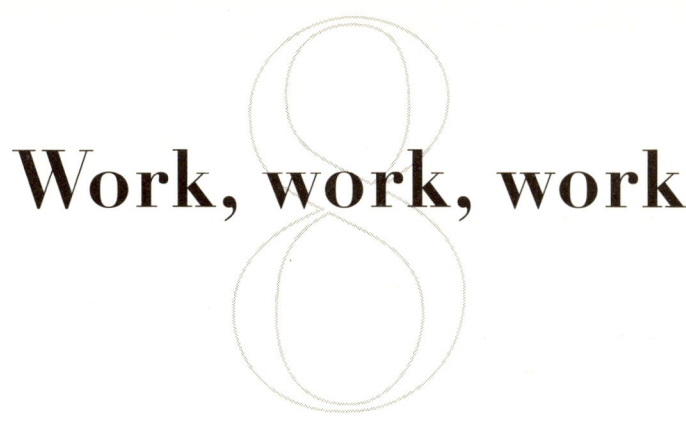

Modern Western culture has conventionally charged men with generating the wages of survival and women with the domestic duties of child-rearing and housekeeping. Although this is now changing in some respects, it forms the legacy we inherited, the burden of the past. For countless men, a commitment to paid work is a social obligation that enables them to feel valued and useful. Men commonly invest emotionally in the role of family 'provider' and seek esteem through public recognition of achievement. In this chapter, we discuss the place of work in the lives of a variety of men.

For example, paid work was central to the lives of men born in the 1920s and 1930s as both the means of survival and the foundation of self-worth. For the elderly men I spoke with, work consisted of demanding physical labour. During the 1940s, they were employed as miners, crane drivers, railway workers, farm labourers, fishermen, factory workers, truck drivers, loggers, barmen, carpenters and electricians. Their working lives were long and arduous.

Hardship and pride

DENIS: I WAS HAPPY WITH MACHINES

Denis was raised in the countryside. After leaving school at the age of 13, he travelled around the local farms and orchards for five years looking for work. He undertook a variety of manual jobs and lived in farm accommodation; when the work was over, he moved on. He had little money and journeyed from job to job on foot or by hitching rides. On one occasion, after a brief spell at a coastal sawmill he heard about work in a mine 80 kilometres inland. After days of walking and hitchhiking, he arrived at the colliery to find that all the jobs been taken. However, he found work wielding a pick and shovel with the railway gangs laying down line in the area. Now 18, he and the other men lived in tents and migrated with the work.

> There were 15 tents and 29 men. I came to the conclusion that all a tent does is keep the dew off you. It doesn't keep rain off or wind, dust, flies, or spiders out. It wasn't much fun, but we got used to it and made our own fun amongst ourselves. (Denis, aged 87)

Inevitably, after two years that job came to an end and the hunt for work began again. He settled for five years in a foundry of the Metal Manufacturing Company. 'It was hard work with 80 lb weights being used sometimes,' he told me. He later returned to the railways as a ganger for three years before coming to rest in the local council's engineering department. Denis began his municipal career as a labourer cleaning out gutters for six months before becoming the driver of a front-end loader. Simultaneously, he decided to run 16 head of cattle 'on the side', so after a five-day week with the council he spent the weekends working on the farm.

> Talk about work, I knew nothing but work, I used to get that tired when I got home, I just couldn't go out to the pictures or anything like that. I was just glad to have a good shower and go to bed. (Denis, aged 87)

Denis continued his working life for another 12 years until 'in the end I got sick, I had a burst ulcer and my doctor told me to take on something less detrimental to my health'. He then transferred to the neighbourhood Parks and Gardens department, where he remained for 11 years until retirement. Denis was particularly content here and took great pleasure in producing colourful displays of flowers that were praised by managers and passers-by alike. Indeed, he took pride in all his work from which he derived considerable satisfaction.

> I was happy with machines. I could make the front-end loader sing. They used to say I could do anything with it. I took my time to do things and never rushed at anything and did it properly. I did take pride in what I'd done. That's the way I work. I work precisely and as neat as possible. (Denis, aged 87)

Nonetheless, on his 40th birthday Denis decided that work was not providing him with sufficient emotional satisfaction and he 'set out to find a wife'. He was married for 37 years but continued to labour hard throughout and work formed the mainstay of our conversation. In this, Denis appears as the archetypical job-oriented man of his era and characteristic of the Diggers.

VICTOR AND STAN: PUTTING UP WITH HARD THINGS

Victor spent 12 arduous and hazardous years diving into the depths to repair fishing nets or patching up the underside of trawlers. It was dangerous work, but it quickly took on a routine quality and he lost his fear: 'I didn't think of it as hard work. I enjoyed it. All I did find hard was that the hours were long' (Victor, aged 75). The next 11 years of his life were filled with equally demanding labour felling logs and driving a crane at the steelworks. Victor took pleasure in showing me a series of merit certificates from the steelworks, observing that work was 'very important to me'.

> You have got to learn how to put up with hard things. You have to have patience, and endure it and do what you can at the time. I have struggled through thick and thin all my life. (Victor, aged 75)

Although these men embraced hard physical work, they also felt its adversities in their bones. Stan (aged 89) repeatedly spoke about work in terms of what had to be 'put up with'. He 'suffered the colliery and lived in a humpy' (a mobile shack). He described farm work as 'a terrible ordeal' and thought of himself as 'lumbering on through a hard working life'. However, despite the hardship he 'took pride' in his work, encapsulating the Digger attitude to life – at least those who avoided the pitfalls of alcohol and gambling. Stan didn't drink or smoke and regarded himself as a 'churchman above all'.

> I'm an individual who can tolerate a lot of hardships and I don't cave in on the first thing that goes mad. I can take the world as it comes, just learn that way. When you're just a boy 18 and now just on 90 that you proved yourself well, you've tolerated the hardships that were served out to you in this hard land. You knew that you'd have hardships no matter, so you'd just have a happy life as you went along. There was no concern for anything else, no good lying down saying 'Oh, what have I got to be happy for?'. I just was happy and doing my own thing. Built my own house and all that sort of caper and never depended on other people to do things for me. I did it myself. (Stan, aged 89)

MODERNITY AND EMOTION MANAGEMENT

A grasp of history helps us to understand why modern men value paid work so highly as a source of pride and pursue it with stoicism and resilience. Our thinking has been shaped by the Enlightenment, a stream of thought associated philosophically with 18th-century writers like Voltaire, Rousseau, Hume and Bacon and socially with the rise of science, capitalism and industrialisation. Here 'reason' was counterposed to emotion in the 'civilising process' and championed as the source of progress for knowledge and society.

Sociologist Norbert Elias[1] suggests that, following the medieval period, modern societies demonstrate a relative shift from external to internal forms of social control that require individuals to 'manage' their emotions. Accordingly, people became subject not only to the overt discipline of the police and law courts, but also shame and embarrassment arose spontaneously in a new way. In other words, the cultural conditions of particular historical periods give rise to specific modes of 'doing emotion'.

In particular, the modern schism of reason and emotion formed along gendered lines, with men associated with rationality and women with feelings. Men's sense of duty and commitment to a work ethic are legacies of Protestantism and the processes of logical calculation associated with capitalism. For example, the factories that sprang up with the industrial revolutions of Europe demanded submission to rigorous discipline. Industries were run according to the clock rather than by the rhythms of nature, requiring social regulation and control of the workforce. Workingmen no longer rose with the morning light and slept with the darkness as country folk had done, but followed the dictate of a timepiece and the clocking-in card. The male factory managers who supervised them functioned through the impersonal task-oriented hierarchical rules of bureaucracy.

The discipline demanded by modern industrial life was achieved not only by external domination but also through a requirement for self-control. Hence, the ways of speaking about men and masculinity that emerged during the 19th and 20th centuries have commanded men to exhibit self-discipline and regulate their emotions. Men have been trained to look outwards to the external world and separated from 'inner' emotion work. It is difficult, then, for men not to be work-oriented control freaks when this is the history they have inherited.

The psychological dynamics of the modern industrial family prepare men to value paid work and public achievement. Boys are encouraged to separate from their mothers more fully than girls and venture out into the external world. This requires the regulation of emotional sensitivities; failure to do so results in sanctions such as being bullied and called a 'mummy's boy'. The necessity for boys to swiftly separate from their mothers generates anxiety and a fragile sense of self.[2] Men become less emotionally independent than women and are more likely to put up psychological defences that promote security. The culturally sanctioned drive for public achievement through work is a dimension of those defences. This is so for contemporary middle-class executives who were born in the 1950s and 1960s as much as for the elderly Diggers.

The emotional compulsion to work

MAURICE: A DRIVE TO WIN

Maurice (aged 37, a senior marketing manager) told me that he was 'a fairly ambitious type of guy' with a 'drive to win and lead people'. He set himself such high benchmarks for success that he was 'never happy with the status quo, even if things are going well' because 'I don't tolerate mediocrity'. Nevertheless, Maurice expressed regret that:

> Sometimes my drive gets in the way of my empathy. Sometimes I think to myself 'Christ, I wish I wasn't as ambitious or as demanding as I am'. I just wish I could let life happen to me and cruise around and not worry – not need to be doing stuff all the time. Diplomacy is sometimes not something I am very good at. (Maurice, aged 37)

Along with personal recognition, corporate success offers considerable financial rewards and, tough-minded though he was, Maurice had the good grace to say that 'looking after two households' was a central motivation for him. However, even Maurice steered clear of the word 'money'. Indeed, there was an evident reticence among these highly paid men to acknowledge the accumulation of wealth as a driving force.

This coyness may have been because they felt an unspoken cultural criticism of their salaries, particularly in conversation with an academic possessing cultural status but lacking financial clout. Nonetheless, I suggest that their reluctance to talk about money also reflected a wish to be understood on a human emotional dimension rather than in terms of their bank balance. After all, these men had agreed to take part in a conversation about their personal lives. They talked about their relationships with parents, wives and children with more ease than they did about their motivation to accrue money.

Most of the executives with whom I spoke shared Maurice's emotional investment in work. Gordon (aged 48) told me that 'work is my biggest driver by far' and that he commonly thought in terms of 'winning and losing'. Likewise, James (aged 49) suggested that he was 'driven to achieve an outcome', while Nick (aged 33) accepted that he was 'overworked and driven. I mean, if you asked people about me they would say overworked and driven and hard and so forth. I think that would come out'.

Nick hedges his account of himself as 'driven' by attributing it to other people, and mitigates even that by only 'thinking' that people would say this. This ambiguity was typical of executive attitudes: there was a powerful commitment to work and yet, like Maurice, there was also an expression of regret or even guilt. They were aware of a growing criticism of 'workaholism' expressed by the women in their lives, which was more marked in their stories than in those of the equally work-oriented but 'pre-feminist' Diggers.

JAMES: CHALLENGES AND SATISFACTIONS

The executives spoke about the emotional satisfaction of overcoming 'challenges' and being 'task-oriented'. James (aged 49) told me that successfully meeting 'managerial challenges' was the cornerstone of his identity.

> I think I have goals, and maybe I did want to please my father when I was younger, but after that it wasn't to please anyone else, but I think it was part of my own self-image. So that is a part of my life, sort of setting challenges and meeting them as best I can ... I've always simply focused on what I'm doing now and doing it well. I am more of a task-oriented person. When there is something to be done, it gets done.
> (James, aged 49)

Language does not simply mirror a pre-given world, but rather gives meaning to it. Our choice of vocabulary is therefore significant because it constitutes the cultural map we navigate with. The selection of words like 'challenges', 'tasks' and 'achievements' speaks of the anonymous object-orientation of businessmen, and about their emotional need for public acknowledgment. Many of the executives called themselves 'people persons' who 'worked through other people' and looked after 'my people'. However, people were grasped through the managerial language of 'task orientation', 'hygiene factors', 'measurement of performance', 'mentoring', 'networking', 'career paths' and so forth. Human beings took on the quality of inanimate objects to be managed and manoeuvred at will. James gave a stark illustration of this when asked about his personal feelings towards the redundancies occurring in his industry.

> Insulated from it. I can't remember a job I've had in the last 20 years where I haven't reduced people; it's just the nature of the task. I simply accept the philosophy that the business, for the business to survive, you've got to make it competitive. If I feel the way that we are doing it is fair, and it is necessary, I'm insulated at the personal level. (James, aged 49)

A 'people person' can be quite selective, then, about the kinds of human beings for whom he feels empathy. The messy lives of living people and their emotional needs can become invisible (or 'reduced') when they are constructed as a component of business. And yet James espoused 'Christian values', was heavily involved in the Church and active in the management of worthwhile community projects. He said it was important 'to have a reference point outside of myself because corporate life is a very narrow existence'. But he nonetheless inhabited a world of self-justifying values that shielded him from the wider consequences of his actions. Indeed, many of the executives overlooked the impact that business demands had on their own families.

Contradictions of work and family

Their jobs made heavy claims upon these executives, including routine 12-hour days, considerable travel and long absences from home. Yet, in their minds they moderated their commitment to work by suggesting that their partners and children were actually more important to them. They frequently reflected on a strange sense of 'How did I get here?' when they discussed the dilemmas of work and family.

GORDON: A SELF-ABSORBED PEOPLE PERSON

Gordon (aged 48) told me: 'The most important thing in my life is family.' However, in literally the very next breath, he suggested: 'Where I have the most value, I believe, is in the work space.'

> If I set out a task, I actually achieve it quite well. So once I'm given a clear, well-defined task I'll invariably accomplish that at the expense of people, I guess. When I look now, I know a lot more about myself and I don't think I actually realised that then but I certainly, um, relationships were there for me to use, not for mutual benefit of individuals. I can look back on that and that was very self-centred and probably extremely aggressive as well in terms of letting out my emotions, and alcohol certainly didn't help that. (Gordon, aged 48)

Here the instrumental goal-centred outlook intrinsic to 'task orientation' is carried over into personal relationships, which are there for his 'use'. His work-oriented life strategy is geared to achieving goals designed to boost his self-esteem at other people's expense. However, Gordon does demonstrate self-awareness and was striving to become a 'people person' who took pride in 'building strong teams'.

Nonetheless, by his own account his wife saw him as a 'dominating influence'. 'As she gets more independent, she sees that as an issue and we have grown apart quite dramatically,' he said. Gordon also spoke of tensions between himself and one of his daughters. 'I find those issues at home far greater in terms of stress than anything I do at work,' he said. But Gordon still saw himself as a family man seeking to achieve a balance between work and home life. He knew that he 'didn't have a great rapport with them' and told me that repairing his relationships with his wife and children was now his main priority. However, he did not address the fact that the 12 hours a day he spent at work might not be helping his cause.

NICK: NEGOTIATION AND AUTHORITY

Providing for their families was the reason executives gave for their intense devotion to work. However, when men work exceptionally long days they inevitably become less physically and emotionally available to those families. For the Digger generation, this was expected, but contemporary women are less accepting of the traditional division of labour. Today, corporate men are in danger of opening up an emotional abyss with their partners that can't be bridged.

Nevertheless, Nick (aged 33, a senior airline financial officer) was not alone in telling me that 'my wife is a willing partner in that process and she takes the lion's share of looking after the face-to-face activity with the children and I am in the background'. These men felt that they were participating in work–home arrangements that at best had been negotiated with their wives, and at worst had their partners' tacit support.

Nick agreed that he worked long hours but added that he and his wife had *discussed* the issue of work and home life regularly. He thought that after four years of dedication to work he would like to assign more time to his family. He recounted his horror that after one long, tiring working day he had snapped at his one-year-old daughter. And yet he suggested that he *did* see his daughter enough and that 'we'll probably get a nanny at some stage and that is the life we have chosen, the professional life. You make your decisions and then you live with them. So we have chosen this life'. Nick's family dialogue took place, it seems, within strategic boundaries that prioritised his working life.

Career-inspired geographical movement inevitably raised issues of negotiation and authority in domestic relationships. Some men consulted their partners, but many made the decision to change jobs before talking to their family. For example, John (aged 48) told his wife: 'Well, I am definitely going to accept this job, I think you ought to come with me.' He recounted that 'she came kicking and screaming'. John regularly moved posts across Australia and Asia to satisfy his need for constant change: 'Every time my wife started getting settled, I'd sort of walk in and say "Well, I've got this job in Indonesia" or wherever. So I enjoyed that kind of change, but it became the thing that pulled us apart; my wife couldn't cope.'

Tony (aged 48, a chief executive officer) told me that all his career changes were negotiated with his wife, and yet he did so ambivalently: 'Every decision I've made, and this may be wrong in hindsight, but I have usually made it with Katherine in 24 hours and she has usually said "Well, if that is what you want to do, just get on with it", you know, she has always been very supportive.' Tony thinks he negotiates with his wife – but he is not entirely sure – and he reveals that negotiations concern Katherine's support for his choices rather than her complete and equal participation in the decision-making.

Individual biographies varied, but tension between executives and their partners was a recurrent theme. At worst, there was outright conflict that led to separation and divorce. At best, there was negotiation that was bounded by the men's ambitions. But one thing the executives agreed on was that their wives needed to be self-reliant with independent lives. Self-sufficient women meant that the work–home fault-line was less fractious. These busy work-oriented men did not necessarily seek old-fashioned subservient and domesticated women. Rather, they wanted homemakers who were *also* socially independent *and* emotionally supportive. Of course, some women may have entered into an unspoken contract by which their husband's absence was exchanged for economic security, a home and children.

Work and children

ALAN: QUALITY TIME WITH THE KIDS

These hardworking executives wanted to be more open and emotionally connected to their children than their fathers had been, and they probably were. And yet, while the desire was there the practice was more circumspect. Alan (aged 47, chief personnel manager) told me that his relationship with his children was 'inadequate from the point of view of time involvement'. He explained that because of the amount of travel he undertook 'the time actually in the home with the kids is pretty limited and that is an issue. It is an issue for us as a couple and for us as a family'. He talked about the 'constant battle' to find more time for his children. A survey by the Institute of Family Studies[3] suggested that 70 per cent of men wish to spend more time with their kids.

Alan thought that since he was often unable to be with his children, 'the time that you do spend with your family has to be quality time'. The notion of 'quality time' is the battle cry of the professional middle class, deployed by parents to justify their excessive working hours. However, it is an idea that has come under increasing scrutiny from child psychologists who suggest that, after all, the *amount* of time spent with children is crucial to their emotional wellbeing. Love is spelt time Alan's wife, who struggled against the all-encompassing nature of his work, was now 'getting less supportive about it as the time goes on, for understandable reasons'.

ANDREW AND GERRY: NOT LIKE MY FATHER?

Andrew (aged 37) was torn between his commitment to work and the emotional pull of his family. His childhood experience of an inexpressive father who never told him that he was loved or spent time with him made this anxiety especially resonant. Andrew reflected mournfully on a father he rarely saw and the lost opportunities to play cricket with him or talk about his feelings. He was aware his wife felt that he worked too hard and had got his priorities askew. He knew he should listen as their relationship was under strain: both were stressed after long days at work and their sex life was in terminal decline. Nonetheless, Andrew remained ambitious and talked about having 'another move or two in me yet'.

> She says that I should be slowing down, I should smell the roses and all this type of thing and your life is passing you by. I say, 'Look, I am trying to build a very sound secure future for yourself and for our son' and I don't want him to go without and this type of thing. (Andrew, aged 37)

Gerry (aged 48) complained that, while his father loved him, he didn't express his affection overtly. He attributed this to 'a mirror of the relationship he may have had with his father; it's different to the one that I share with my children'. Gerry appreciated that changes have occurred in father–child relationships since the Digger generation. Nevertheless, his own children protested the amount of time he spent at work. In fairness, Gerry did not simply give lip service to his family's needs. When his children were young, he played regularly with them and today he and his wife stage a weekly dinner for extended family and friends. Nonetheless, he was compelled by his social environment to make choices that isolated him from loved ones. Even when a man is committed to his family, there are forces at work that push him in another direction.

Gerry and other executives were taught to be ambitious, hardworking men by childhood families with conventional gender relationships.

They understand that family roles have now changed and that men are asked (and usually want) to be more emotionally involved with their children. Nevertheless, career ambition compels them to make choices that disallow their own stated aspirations. They are committed to being well-paid determined members of the corporate community, which by its nature limits family time.

Individualism in Western culture

The relationship dilemmas faced by executives are not unique; rather, they are a particular instance of cultural tensions between individualism and mutual aid. The compulsion to become a unique person with a successful career collides with our growing obligation to put more time and effort into relationships. And the emphasis given to individual accomplishment (usually measured in financial terms) generates substantial pressure to 'succeed', creating the conditions for self-absorption and social isolation.

We are too often obsessed with what we want and how we will get it at the expense of connecting with other human beings. Yet, it is our relationships with other people that support happiness. By emphasising individual accomplishment, we generate its dark shadow – a sense of personal failure. Rampant individualism and its spouse social isolation are the indifferent parents of depression (see chapter 6).

In contrast, evidence suggests that cultures which emphasise social solidarity experience fewer mental health problems than societies oriented towards individuals. Depression is higher in the individualistic and competition-oriented Western world than elsewhere. Psychologist John F Shumaker claims that clinical depression hardly exists in non-Western cultures that offer its members social support and collective ritual ways to deal with loss.[4]

THE PROCESSES OF INDIVIDUATION

Individualism cannot be explained simply by resort to genetic programming; on the contrary, current thinking in evolutionary biology stresses sociability as the key to human survival. Rather, the practices of culture create individuals as we understand them. The institutions of our societies are geared to individuals rather than collectives, addressing us as consumers rather than citizens. We are urged to take 'personal responsibility' for our health, our education, our financial future, our careers, and our beliefs. Above all, we are expected to 'make the most' of our lives and be 'successful' individuals. Hardly a week goes by without a Sunday newspaper magazine telling us how to achieve as individuals.

We can no longer rely on the state or the Church or a collective culture to make our life choices. These institutions are unable to provide the stories of our lives and their preordained paths, as they once did. Ours is a society in which we must decide for ourselves what to do, how to act and who to be. We must sustain our own story about the past and project a desired future. Today, tensions between personal freedom and commitment to others, concerning say work and family, are thrown into sharp relief.

MY PARADOXICAL INDIVIDUALISM

Like all of us, I am a child of my time. The most influential period of my cultural formation was the late 1960s and its extension into the mid-1970s, which I spent in Cambridge (UK). Here I encountered students, 'hippie' culture, and the New Left politics of protest. These were the heady days of anti-Vietnam War demonstrations, the Campaign for Nuclear Disarmament, the emergence of contemporary feminism, talk of cultural revolution, and a rejection of the protestant work ethic. This was the crucible in which many of my social and political attitudes were forged; including a sense that paid work is not the purpose of life and that ethics of social justice should prevail over individual aggrandisement.

There is a paradox at the heart of 'sixties culture' that I embody; on the one hand, we rejected individualism in favour of collective politics, and yet we were intensely individualistic in asserting our difference from mainstream parental culture. We set out to be culturally distinct in our music, clothes and relationship to work and money. Although many of the so-called baby boomer generation were politically motivated (as was I), we tended to prioritise our individual freedom and 'personal growth'.

While I do hold many of the 'radical' collective impulses of the 1960s, I am also aware that I have acted in self-centred ways that caused suffering to myself and others (see chapter 9).

My Left-hippie impulses led me to reject the pursuit of career and the accumulation of money for its own sake. I have also been opposed to, and often in conflict with, the hierarchical structures of organisations in which I have worked. I don't take kindly to the inevitable attempts that organisational managers make to control me. Perhaps in every manager I see my authoritarian father. In any case, I have wanted to plough my own furrow. However, this has also meant that I have not always been overly co-operative with my immediate co-workers either (but I am getting better), even in political resistance to the strategies of managements. I am aware that, even as I write books that profess a politics of equality, social justice and liberation, I am simultaneously in pursuit of personal acclamation. I would say that personal relationships are more important to me than work, but I have devoted considerable time to writing!

My pursuit of autonomous self-development has enriched a life that has not been without its accomplishments; reading, thinking and writing has its personal and cultural value. However, my drive towards individual achievement at work is founded on a self-critical voice that has simultaneously fuelled a struggle with depression. My quest for attainment has been sustained by a recurrent feeling of being not quite 'good enough'. I also suffered from the social isolation that individualism brings: when I fell into the abyss, there was no one there to catch me. One of the lessons I learnt from depression is the need to spend more time with people and less time committed to work. I have become more sociable than I once was. And it works. I am much happier.

Paradoxically, this shift to a more relational stance has come through personal self-reflection. The individualism of our culture is a double-edged sword: it threatens to condemn us to self-absorption, but it generates possibilities of making ourselves anew. This is the era of 'working on oneself' (see chapter 11), which enables us to self-consciously change our life path and reassess our commitments.

MATTHEW'S GONE SURFING

A year after I talked with Matthew, I heard that he had left the pharmaceutical company where he worked as a human resources manager to go on a worldwide surfing trip. I was pleased for him because he had done what he had hoped to do. Matthew had told me that he 'just went down the whole career path; undergraduate, postgraduate, get a job, try and climb the ladder and all that sort of stuff' (Matthew, aged 29). He studied politics and then human resources management because he was interested in 'power relationships'. Having been in some badly managed organisations, he felt that he could do better: 'I felt I should put my money where my mouth is, you know.'

However, Matthew's career did not work out as he had hoped. Human resource management did not give him the satisfaction that he expected. He found that he was continually 'moving deckchairs on the *Titanic*', unable to exert any significant influence on the companies' management. Further, he was now working 12-hour days, which prevented him from developing other valued dimensions of his life. 'It's a bit of a letdown and that was very disappointing,' he said. 'After working all those hours and expecting all these wonderful things to happen and they didn't. And the choice was either to get incredibly disappointed about that or to focus on getting rewards in life from other directions.' He wisely chose the latter.

A recurrent theme of my conversation with Matthew was his values. Values tell us what something is worth, what we aspire to and what we are willing to do; they provide us with the crucial signposts of our lives. 'I think the most fundamental value is to be at peace with yourself and that comes from doing things which are in accordance with your values,' he said. However, Mathew was struggling with a realisation that he was prioritising work over other important dimensions of his life, but had found it 'hard to give up the image of myself as a successful person'. He was also concerned about working in an industry with questionable ethics: he worried that pharmaceutical companies continually put their profits before the needs of people and specifically that they were withholding vital HIV-treatment drugs from poorer countries. This troubled him because he felt that happiness was the outcome of acting in accordance with one's values, and he doubted that he was doing so.

Matthew had been practising meditation, becoming 'a big fan of sitting still and having no noise for half an hour a day'. He had decided to make more space for meditation, surfing and jazz guitar in his life.

> I had to say to myself, 'Do you really want to keep on climbing this ladder and work longer and longer hours and have less and less time to yourself or do you want to go and do things which are outside of work, which builds your life in a different way?', and I have decided to go down that track. (Matthew, aged 29)

Crumbling relationships

In our mother-centred families, women generally carry out the emotional sustenance of children. Fathers are more involved in paid work and 'doing' things; they are often more emotionally distant from their children. A consequence is that boys become men who, like their fathers, want to go out into the world to make their mark. The association our culture forges between men, work and the celebration of individual achievement strengthens this orientation.

Accordingly, the Diggers from the rest home had lived lives focused on work and military duty. The executives too had a powerful emotional identification with worldly success. Not only had family and school taught them a powerful work ethic, but also they enjoyed public acclaim. Being driven to succeed, these men struggled to find a balance between their emotional connections with their family and the demands of working life. They faced a good deal of criticism from their wives and children about this and they expressed regret that work so often subtracted from their personal lives.

Nevertheless, these men continued to devote most of their time to pursuing individual success at work. As dedicated individuals, they are the product of a culture that compels them to do so. Paradoxically, this individualism also enables men to reflect on their lives and change their path. Often, the impulse to do this comes from personal dissatisfaction with crumbling relationships, which is the theme of our next chapter.

Men and relationships

PETER IN LOVE

Peter is the 45-year-old managing director of a retail company. Encouraged by the high expectations of his middle-class parents, Peter devoted much of his early life to study and work. Then, during his forties, he unexpectedly fell in love. His maturity made him unusually reflective about his feelings, which show emotion to be a complex mix of physical feelings and cultural interpretation.

> Often when I was driving to work I would get this strange fluttery feeling in my body. My arms and legs felt weird and slightly shaky. But they weren't. I felt apprehension in my chest and stomach. Anyway, I didn't know why. It took me a while to decide that it was my anticipation at seeing Melanie rather than my normal anxieties about work. (Peter, aged 45)

Human emotions are an outcome of neurological functioning and our conscious awareness of it. A brain that can then classify its experience linguistically generates a universe distinct from one that cannot. The difference between anticipation and anxiety, or apprehension and excitement, is not simply intensity of bodily sensation but the way we interpret them.

> When I met Melanie, I was immediately attracted to her but the funny thing was it was more her voice than anything else. It was soothing. It made me feel sexy and safe at the same time. Then there was all the anticipation and excitement of going out together and wondering what was going to happen and hoping, of course, but not wanting to hope too much in case, you know, to avoid disappointment … One day it just slipped out and I said 'I love you'. I immediately felt anxious and stupid, but lucky for me she responded. That changes everything. Everything seemed to shift a gear. All the things I had been feeling and wondering about came together and it was obvious. I was in love. (Peter, aged 45)

Cognition, physiological response and cultural naming processes constitute a circuit of interacting elements necessary to the generation of an emotion. Peter's experience of love engages 'unconscious' feelings of sexual attraction based on *electro-biochemical* activity that is explained by *evolutionary* processes of mating and bonding. However, love and attraction also entail conscious *cognitive* processes. Perhaps when he first met Melanie, Peter was thinking 'Wow, she's gorgeous' or 'I like her', thoughts that were accompanied by embodied feelings of arousal – the jittery body and the beating heart.

Peter acted on those feelings in *culturally* accepted ways. He asked her out. They went out for dinner, talked, held hands, kissed and eventually 'slept together'. Love was then named in words. The process of speaking together about love triggered further physiological feelings, conscious cognitions (for example, the ethical considerations that are essential to love) and culturally appropriate expressions of 'love' (they married).

Human beings are social animals, we thrive in the context of positive human relationships and we wither in isolation. Like Peter and Melanie, we all seek love and human connection. Available research on happiness concludes that the richer one's social life, the happier one is (see chapter 11). It is no accident that solitary confinement is a severe punishment and that loneliness is at the core of depression (see chapter 6). The more isolated one is, the more one is vulnerable to despair.

Friendship and isolation

Feelings of isolation are common among men. Michael (aged 47), a men's movement activist, suggested that this is why 'men's groups' exist. 'We all have this isolation thing,' he said. Men attend men's groups to be listened to, as Graham explained:

> Three of us who were friends started talking and there seems to be the need to be a friends ingredient in men's work because our stuff is about isolation so deeply that, unless there is a genuine person-to-person relationship, the work is barely possible at all. Isolation and abuse are the two big men's issues, so every guy presents with some version of isolation or abuse, of himself or someone else. (Graham, aged 45)

Social isolation is a condition that all denizens of the 21st century face as families and communities fall apart. Nevertheless, loneliness has its specific causes and conditions for men, who tend to be more interpersonally competitive than women. Men often miss out on the preparation for relationships that women receive, learning instead to seek individual solutions to problems. Men are often too busy working to give sufficient time and energy to their relationships.

TONY AND GERARD: BUSILY ALONE

In chapter 6, we saw that isolation was both root and fruit of Ben's depression and drug addiction; and loneliness lay behind the alcoholism suffered by Eddy and my father. But social seclusion also impacts on the lives of busy middle-class executives. 'I don't really have any friends here. I have a lot of colleagues, lots of acquaintances, but I don't have any bosom pals,' said chief executive officer Tony (aged 48). He had joined a support group for CEOs because 'there's not many people you can talk to, which is very true, which is one of the challenges actually'.

> There is always something more to be done in business to keep you busy, so trying to stop and find time for mates or family is tough. Then you discover that you haven't got any friends anyway to go out with and your wife is the only person you talk to, really talk to. And that scares me

a bit because it's like all your eggs in one basket, too much pressure. (Tony, aged 48)

Senior telecommunications executive Gerard lived alone in Sydney and bemoaned the fact his married colleagues had wives to act as their 'social administrators'. He understood that the heavy demands of work meant that 'trying to make regular arrangements to meet up with friends is important'. However:

> My behaviour is, I think, fairly classic male behaviour in that I can let things slip for quite a long time and the combination of living by myself and a demanding job mean that you can go for, you can find yourself getting into patterns where you're working and not doing a whole lot else and then you have to try and arrest that. (Gerard, aged 36)

Interestingly, in an age of globalisation when work makes increasing demands on our time, Sydney-based Gerard was building a relationship with a woman in Los Angeles. The paradox of seeking closeness with somebody at great distance seems emblematic of our times.

The absence of friendship networks was a striking feature of executive lives. Perhaps the modern middle-class culture of work is more isolating than the bygone world of working-class Diggers, who more commonly used the pronoun 'we': 'we were captured', 'we were put in Changi prison', 'we suffered more than the Japanese'. A repeated motif of Diggers' talk was the value of their mates. Denis is talking here about the hardship of working on the railways:

> It wasn't much fun, but we got used to each other and made our own fun amongst ourselves. Different things would happen that made you laugh if you'd care to listen to them. It was hard living, but we were young and didn't care. We used to go to dances; some couldn't go because they didn't have money or clothes. They used to borrow clothes from us. Every time there was a dance, some would say, 'Oh, how about a loan of your trousers'. We were broke, but we used to put our money into our clothes so that we could go to dances together. (Denis, aged 87)

The world of work and war offered Denis's generation greater social contact with other men than is the case today. Work has become more competitive, individualistic and less collective than it once was, particularly for middle-class executives. However, because the pub was an important place in which to make their connections, these elderly men exhibited significant levels of alcoholism (see chapter 7). While their experience of male friendship at work diverged, the executives and old soldiers did share a focus on sexual relationships as a route out of isolation.

Women and marriage

Heterosexual men often rely on women for friendship and emotional support. This was certainly the case for the socially isolated executives. 'She is my best friend, she's the only one I talk to. I haven't got a best friend that I talk to,' said Maurice (aged 48). Marriage is positively correlated with greater levels of self-reported life satisfaction[1] and evidence suggests that married men are more emotionally secure than singles.[2] But, sadly, divorce statistics suggest that marriage is not always a happy experience for men or women.

MARRIAGE AND ME

My own experience of marriage has been complex and troubled. I have been married and divorced three times, which is two marriages and three divorces more than I would have wanted. This is not the place to recount the specific details of each marriage. Further, while the women and I all played our parts, I am only going to discuss myself; and I do not have a full explanation of events. However, along with other men, my emotional reliance on women played its part.

My childhood anxiety (see chapters 4 and 5) followed me into adulthood and I looked to women to provide me with sanctuary. I asked marriage to fulfil its promise of emotional security. Men often evaluate relationships through the optics of sexuality, so when I felt my first two marriages were not physically sustaining, I experienced loss and desertion. I then sought the solutions for my discomfort in the obvious self-defeating fashion, relationships with other women. I felt my third marriage to be of a different order; for me, it was an intimate bond on which to build a world. However, during this ten-year marriage I suffered from repeated bouts of deep depression, which undermined our relationship.

Subsequently, I learnt to supply myself with emotional support through self-soothing. A successful relationship depends on us validating ourselves before we can expect that others will hold our hand. Rather than allow other people to determine our worth, we have first to see ourselves as valuable. I now understand that I should not rely on one person to fulfil my emotional needs, as many men do. But as the stories of the Diggers testify, tensions between self-reliance, emotional security and dependency are not unique to me.

The Diggers: A story of tradition

'Naturally, as age went on I happened to get married,' said 89-year-old Stan. Sadly, his wife passed away after only three years of wedlock – 'she just caved in and died' – and he never married again. And herein lies a wider theme of love and loss. All but one of the Diggers had married and suffered loss courtesy of death and/or divorce. Eight of the 20 men had sustained long-term marriages with one partner who later died. Nine of them had married, divorced and then remarried. Two men married but their wives died shortly after the wedding and they did not remarry. The one man who had never been married said that sex and romance had played very little part in his life.

LASTING MARRIAGES

Jenny and Victor met at a local dance and continued with their shared pastime throughout their marriage. Jenny was only 16 when she proposed to the 25-year-old Victor. They were married the following year, producing a son and a daughter. Victor told me that life together created 'a very happy family'. Edward came home from the war weak and 'shattered'. Since he and his wife had not been together for nearly six years, life was not going to be easy. They faced considerable economic hardship, he had endured a Japanese POW camp and they were unable to have the children they wanted. Yet, 'it was our life together; we just simply started again where we left off'. They remained contentedly married for 55 years, which ended only with her death.

'I have had a hard life in my young stages,' said Alan (aged 79), 'but me married life was real good up until the sickness of my wife'. He considered marriage to be the most valuable dimension of his entire life. Of course, they had 'little tiffs, like, that sort of thing', but 'I can say that I have lived a good married life. I met the right girl at the right time and she turned out to be a nice woman and we got on all right'. They were married for 39 years until her death.

The personal qualities of women are obviously a major factor in the constitution of happy lasting marriages. Nevertheless, there are shared characteristics among these men. The most significant commonality was their stable childhood homes, where they acquired the habitual ways of intimacy. They knew what it was to love and be loved. Victor was 'treasured by his parents' and cherished them in return. Edward had a 'good dad' and 'a nice' mother who formed a 'happy family life' for him. Alan's parents separated when he was 11, but shared the parenting, minimalising his distress and demonstrating that love is what children need rather than the precise family form in which it occurs.

Since neither Victor nor Edward were drinkers, and alcohol played only 'a moderate part' in Alan's life, they avoided the destructive role of alcohol in their relationships (see chapter 7). These men took a constructive outlook on life's problems. Their minds were taken up with the optimistic self-talk associated with contentment rather than the flow of negative thoughts that generates depression (see chapter 6).

Despite the difficulties they faced, Edward and his wife 'just counted our blessings as we were'. They were supported by their Christian faith and 'just got on with life'. Alan and Victor spoke positively about their wives being 'marvellous', 'a good wife' and a 'nice person'. These men also took pride in their paid work, which is suggestive of a wider care for themselves and their partners. They valued a job done well for its own sake and not simply for the money. In short, emotionally stable, balanced and self-reliant men sustain long-term marriages in what is no doubt a mutually reinforcing process.

PROBLEM MARRIAGES

Less balanced men often swing between feelings of grandiosity and inadequacy. When we win at sport, gain that sought-after promotion or fall in love, we receive praise and validation from others. We feel like kings of the world. But the high is short-lived and we are compelled to repeat the performance, which is never enough. If we cannot achieve our ambitions or if we lose the support of others, we are quickly deflated. The 'dark' side of a life directed towards external validation is the need to take flight from constant self-interrogation. Am I good enough? Have I done well enough? Am I worthy to be loved?

When relationships were unable to shore up their fragile defences, some Diggers sought relief through compulsive behaviours (addictions). Since love, intimacy and feelings of self-worth are heavily tied to sexual activity for men, so the demise of their sex life was felt as abandonment. A troubled feature of the more thorny relationships was the intensification of this loss by alcohol. The damage inflicted by drinking and gambling was then a significant cause of marital breakdown.

ERIC: SHE DENIED ME LOVE

Eric was raised in 'quite a distant family' in which his father used violence as a means of discipline: 'We got the stock whip. He didn't mess around. That was the old way' (Eric, aged 83). Eric was not close to his father or his siblings, but did maintain a warm relationship with his mother. Already an emotionally sensitive and apprehensive man, Second World War military service was particularly challenging for Eric: 'Most of it was kept inside because you didn't know when it was gonna be you.' On his return, traumatised and in search of emotional comfort, Eric took up with the first woman to show any interest in him. They married after only two months of knowing each other, when she proposed to him.

Eric and his wife were married for 37 years, during which time 'she gave me two lovely kids'. However, 'I was unhappy for years because she denied me sex. She denied me love, she denied me everything. I took it for years.' Eric felt cheated, lonely and unloved. In order to deal with these distressing feelings, he spent more and more time at work and in the pub. Arguments ensued about his absentee drinking, until he eventually packed his suitcase and left home. He then spent even more time working and drinking. He was devastated when retirement was forced upon him and, left without purpose, he again sought solace at the bar.

A harsh family environment and a hard-nosed father led Eric to identify love with women. In particular, affection was associated with sex. After the trauma of war, he sought comfort in the arms of a woman but felt abandoned when their sex life deteriorated. Eric then substituted work, mateship and alcohol for the intimacy he had hoped for with his wife. Eric reminds me of my father; a sensitive man who, disturbed by war, sought solace first in a marriage, and then, failing to find it there, in anaesthetic intoxication.

When men are faced with the loss of emotional security that a sexual relationship was meant to provide, they commonly get angry. A cyclical process then ensues, because women often seek intimacy as a prerequisite of sexual activity and so respond to male anger by retreating further. Men and women can then become involved in an escalating spiral of mutual pain. But there is always the hope that we can begin anew.

PHIL: A SECOND CHANCE

During his first marriage, Phil also experienced sex as the means and medium for his exclusion. 'That was a disaster, really. It had me right down,' said Phil (aged 77). 'You couldn't feel outward, you couldn't feel spontaneous with her. She shut you out because it wasn't her way.' Indeed, sex was not even a topic of conversation that Phil's first wife would engage in.

Fortunately, Phil was able to find long-lasting emotional satisfaction with his second wife Mary. After her death, which was a terrible blow, he remained close to her children, who continue to visit him. As he said: 'It's the feeling that they give you, you sort of feel that they want to do these things with you and I want to see them.' However, not all the Diggers were able to forge positive connections with their stepchildren. Some marriages were torn apart by the complexities of reconstituted families, notably parenting the children from their wives' previous relationships.

Harold's second marriage foundered over jealousy of his wife's children. Retrospectively, he views those feelings as groundless, but at the time he resented the attention they received: 'I got into drink and I had bouts of bad temper, which up until then had been foreign to my nature.'

A story about 'lasting' and 'problem' marriages grossly simplifies the complexity of men's lives. The 'good' and the 'bad' are but archetypes representing the poles of a continuum that encompasses all kinds of messy in-betweens. But, the theme I want to highlight is this: men need love and intimacy. The more a secure childhood has equipped them with emotional stability, the more they are able to skilfully give and receive love. In the absence of such security, fear and anxiety fill the space. This leads to an emotional 'neediness' and dependence on women that paradoxically pushes intimacy away. Where intimacy and love are absent, workaholism, alcohol abuse and violence provide ways to cope with emotional suffering.

Since women's ways of conducting relationships are not always skilful either, we should avoid pathologising men. Nonetheless, the traditional social and economic power of men, which shaped the character of marriage, works against intimacy. It is difficult to have a close loving relationship with someone over whom you claim superiority or to respond lovingly as a woman when you feel dominated. Happily, the character of contemporary relationships is now changing in ways that may allow love and intimacy to flourish.

The emergence of emotional democracy

Throughout human history, men have occupied positions of economic, social and political power. It is largely men who have been monarchs, prime ministers, captains of industry, doctors and professors. Men have also claimed legal and financial leadership over the family. However, our cultural expectations of relationships are being transformed. In particular, we can no longer rely on the Church, the state or the extended family to hold a marriage together. The law has been making divorce easier to obtain and most people don't believe that ending a marriage is sinful. In an era of individual consumer choice, from mobile phones to medicine, we now need reasons to continue a relationship.

Today, our justifications for maintaining a relationship have to be constructed in the light of women's claim to equality. Women are increasingly unwilling to accept the conventional domestic division of labour and men's emotional dependence on them. They wish to participate in business, in the arts, as politicians and as co-contributors to family decision-making. Women have pioneered radical changes in the emotional order that have shaken the taken-for-granted practices of male authority. It is not enough for women that the family be a social arrangement, as it has been for much of human history, in which they provide domestic duties and sex in exchange for economic survival. Women want relationships of love, care and justice in which they are valued as unique people.

Popular psychology provides widespread authoritative support for democratising love relationships. Self-help books stress the importance of dialogue, negotiation and emotional openness in preserving partnerships. Research suggests that the capacity to perceive and accurately distinguish our feelings, the ability to understand and reason about emotions, and the competence to effectively regulate them, are features of happier marriages.[3] For relationships to sustain themselves today, we must recognise that our partner is sad or angry and be able to talk without being caught up in a defensive rage. We need to be able to let go of our resentments, or at least to express them appropriately.

Our emphasis on individual choice, combined with women's march towards social equality and the diffusion of psychological thinking, is generating the conditions for greater emotional democracy.[4] This entails accomplishing relationships within an environment of moral equality. For contemporary relationships to survive without binding by law or tradition, they must involve respect for personal autonomy, trust, reciprocity and equality. Emotional democracy requires participants to develop the skills to perceive, understand, express and regulate emotion in order to negotiate the conduct of relationships. Self-validation and wise personal emotion management are required for discussion to occur between independent equals.[5]

The inequality once intrinsic to family life is no longer inevitable or desirable. Women are no longer the property of men, nor are marriages primarily economic arrangements. Essential to the relatively recent idea of a 'relationship' is the expectation of intimacy based on shared communication. This emerging expectation of family life is one that men cannot ignore if their relationships are to endure. Nor can they afford to be over-reliant on women for emotional support, or they risk finding themselves divorced and alone. Yet, men's relationship to emotional democracy appears ambivalent.

Men, women and relationships

A study by British sociologists Jean Duncombe and Dennis Marsden[6] suggests that men think of relationships as occurring between separate parallel people. They seek a *life in common* with their wives that includes domestic comforts and psychological support; but not intimacy, dialogue and self-awareness. In contrast, their wives want *a common life* with an empathetic partner including an exchange of emotional familiarity. Duncombe and Marsden describe substantial dissatisfaction among women with the inability of men to engage in emotional intimacy, and with the priority they give to work.

A report by the Human Rights and Equal Opportunities Commission suggests that women continue to perform 90 per cent of child-care tasks and 70 per cent of all family work.[7] Duncombe and Marsden report that most wives accepted inequality in domestic tasks as being counterbalanced by their husbands' work demands. However, they expressed deep disappointment with imbalances in emotional exchange: they felt they tenderly reassured their husbands, but their partners failed to reciprocate. Wives who perceived their marriages as conforming to the ideal of emotional companionship often excused the unequal distribution of domestic tasks.

Men often respond to women's desire for more emotional communication with incomprehension, say Duncombe and Marsden. Some try to avoid discussions or become angry. Others seek to 'win' clashes by using cool and articulate arguments that evade emotional engagement. Men said they did have feelings, but were reluctant to disclose them. The report's authors comment that emotional concerns are becoming an increasing source of friction as the pressures towards emotional communication transform marriage. They suggest that men's disinclination to express intimate emotions contributes to relationship troubles and family breakdown.

THE CLASH OF WORK AND INTIMACY

Although the broad brushstrokes of this story are recognisable, it relies on cultural stereotypes, overlooking men who are able to speak openly about their emotions. I talked to men whose capacity to develop emotional self-awareness through dialogue was far greater than Duncombe and Marsden suggest. Many men are aware of the pressures towards emotional democracy in relationships, but feel pulled apart by the contradictory demands of intimacy and work.

Many of the executives spoke about the need for dialogue and equality with their partners. They expressed a wish to be more involved as fathers with their children. A few were putting these words into practice; and many said they were frustrated by the lack of opportunity that the demands of paid employment allowed. They felt that it was in the best interests of their families for them to be committed to well-remunerated work (see chapter 8).

A recent survey[8] found that lack of time together was the single biggest obstacle (named by 38 per cent of respondents) to successful partnerships. Thirty per cent of respondents working full-time wished to alter their working arrangements to achieve a better work–family balance. There is change afoot in contemporary relationships, with more men talking about shared and negotiated relationships, though a gap between rhetoric and practice remains.

Derek (aged 49, a health service manager) told me he was a shy, anxious person who became 'emotionally detached' from his wife and children during periods of family tension. Feeling that his commitment to work 'was out of balance', he could see 'a real risk for me having so few friends and having my wife as not just my best friend but in a sense my *only* close friend'. He understood the need to change his behaviour for the wellbeing of himself and his family, but he was not always able to do so. This was a tension felt by all the executives.

FRANK'S AMBIVALENT ATTITUDE

The high-flying managers I spoke with said that they valued human relationships and sought to negotiate with their partners. They said that they treasured the 'precious moments of family time' (Frank, aged 43, managing director of a pharmaceutical company) and understood that men could no longer take women for granted. Yet, they spent much of their time and energy at work.

> I discussed recently with my father that the expectations from mothers today, or let's say wives, is much greater than it was; there is no question about it. I mean, my father didn't travel but he did work crazy hours and my mother would, whatever time he came home, my mother would cook his meal then and I know parents of other kids of a different generation where the mother would prepare the suitcase and accept anything, at least in public, would accept anything that would happen. Whereas these days, probably rightly so, it wouldn't happen. (Frank, aged 43)

Frank reveals an ambivalence about gender relations that was widespread. On the one hand, he accepts that greater autonomy for women is right and proper. But on the other hand, he expresses nostalgia for a time when women's expectations of men were lower. Frank's sense of gender justice is subsequently hedged by the word 'probably'. These corporate men did understand that the world of male–female relationships was changing and that they needed to adapt. They said they were willing to live differently from their parents and were participants in the complex processes of negotiating personal life. They told me this during a well-earned break in their 12-hour working day.

Executives had mastered the vocabulary of greater emotional openness, talking about democratic relationships in genuine and heartfelt ways. However, their commitment to emotional democracy was almost always bounded by the constraints of working life. They were not yet willing or able to change the parameters of work in order to prioritise their relationships. In circular fashion, these men were the product of a society that produced work-oriented men who then made choices that reproduced that very same pattern again, though with some variations. Nevertheless, the adoption of at least the language of gender equality and shared emotional life does indicate that something is changing in the universe of corporate man.

THE CHANGING FAMILY

The tensions between men and women are taking their toll on marriage. The Institute of Family Studies[9] notes that in 2001 a couple with children constituted only 35.7 per cent of families, a 20 per cent decline since 1976. Couples do represent the majority of families in which children live, though 10.7 per cent of families with a child under 18 are now 'blended families'. A third of all marriages now consist of at least one person who has been married before. Single-parent families are becoming more common, rising from 7.1 per cent of families with dependent children in 1969 to 22.3 per cent in 2003. Almost 27 per cent of children spend some time before they are 18 living in a single-parent family.

For some commentators, these developments represent the 'decline of the family', which is held responsible for a range of social problems including poor educational achievement, crime and violence. However, the conventional 1950s two-parent family was itself the site of violence, the subordination of women, child abuse and 'mental illness'. While the instability of the family poses problems for emotional wellbeing, especially for children, it may also be heralding increasingly egalitarian relationships. Men may not be embracing this as swiftly as women, but there is movement. Some men are undergoing a period of self-examination that may assist in the development of new kinds of relationship.

Men looking in the mirror

All of the participants in the 'men's movement' with whom I spoke had been married. Seven of ten had subsequently been divorced and formed new relationships. Two of the three men who had remained married complained of not having had sex with their wives for many years. Relationships, then, were an important issue for these men. It was Glen's (aged 50) concerns about male–female sexual relationships that drew him into 'men's activities'. He started to organise groups so that he could have someone to talk with about intimacy. This was not possible with women, he said, because his 'desperate need for sex' stood in the way. He suggested that men use sex to cope with their loneliness. 'Sex comforts men deeply,' he told me, to the point of addiction.

MIKE: LETTING GO OF FEAR

Mike's changing relationships with women represent the kind of 'personal growth' that the psychologically oriented wing of the 'men's movement' advocates. His first marriage had folded because of his jealousy and aggression. Mike then entered a period of 'deep deep depression' in response to his long-term feelings of abandonment. He found that meditation helped him deal with despair and led him to a new understanding of himself. He came to appreciate that his own insecurity pushed him to control women through anger and violence: 'I was able to see myself clearly for the first time and I didn't like what I saw.'

An engagement with 'spirituality' and the 'men's movement' enabled Mike to begin a protracted process of refashioning himself: 'Through assiduous work I was able to slowly modify how I expressed my fears and frustrations and my anger, control my anger.' Mike told me that his childhood insecurities had led him to seek solace with women while simultaneously spawning the fear that his needs would not be met. He learnt that by 'letting go of my expectations about how my wife is going to relate to me there is less disappointment and less disappointment leads to less fear and then she is able to feel warmer towards me'. Ironically, in his current marriage he feels that 'I am the articulate one who is in touch with his feelings and she's the quiet one who doesn't really express her feelings very well or communicate very well'.

RICHARD: LEARNING FROM PAST MISTAKES

Richard contributed to the demise of his relationships with women, but not through an unwillingness to talk. Instead, anxiety, self-absorption and poor emotional management were the culprits. He was willing and able to *talk* about emotions, but this was not enough; he also needed to listen.

Richard's emotional insecurities led him to marry the first woman to show any sexual interest. Since he felt unloved and unlovable, he swiftly attached himself to anyone willing to hold him. Ironically, the swift demise of their sex life and with it his emotional security led him to abandon the relationship. A short-term 'affair' was then followed by a 16-year marriage that included two children. Richard felt that in many ways this marriage had been a success. It had lasted a number of years and the children, with whom he still had regular contact, had coped well with divorce. Nevertheless, it was now his turn to be abandoned, a factor in his oncoming depression.

The introspection of psychotherapy, men's groups and meditation encouraged a self-awareness that aided Richard's recovery from despair. In particular, 'I found a greater self-acceptance,' he said.

> I am much calmer, much more in control than I used to be. I don't let things get to me quite as much as I did. There was a lot of anger and anxiety that I think prompted the depression. I can see them more clearly now and so I am able to kind of distance myself from them. Stand back and look at them more carefully so they don't get a grip on me. It doesn't always work, but mostly it does. I have always been able to talk, but now I can listen more as well and talk more carefully. I think my current relationship is benefiting from that enormously. (Richard, aged 46)

'Men can learn from past mistakes,' Richard concluded. He discovered that just listening to his new partner and not trying to solve every problem was an important skill. 'I felt it my responsibility to fix everything,' he said. 'I think as men, generally speaking, we want to do that and a lot of the complaints that women have about men these days centre around that sort of stuff. Often, they just want to be heard and have their feelings acknowledged.' Today he is clear that he doesn't want a relationship just to meet his sexual needs, but wants 'intimacy and friendship'.

Mark (aged 50) had learnt a similar lesson. He had been a very goal-oriented planner 'bordering on the workaholic', which had caused difficulties for his relationships. However, with each new partnership, 'I think I am learning each time; I do a bit better each time, I think'. The key difference 'each time' was the increased level of emotional communication in the relationship and a 'letting go of the need to be in control'. He told me that his current long-standing marriage worked because he had learnt to communicate better. He put his earlier marital breakups down to 'mismatched expectations', explaining that the discomforts of disintegrating relationships had taught him to listen more carefully.

SIMON: SEEKING A MORE BALANCED PATH

Participation in men's groups is not a prerequisite for seeking new ways to conduct relationships. While the commitment of executives to paid work was often detrimental to their relationships, Simon (aged 39) was the standout exception. He thought himself a 'fish out of water' in the office because of his dislike of team sport and inclination to prioritise his family over work. Simon trained as a lawyer and was now in a senior advisory position with an international IT company. He told me of a childhood spent in a loving family of Italian heritage with little money. He had been taught at state schools and worked to pay for his tertiary education. Socially, he felt 'like an outsider' among what he called the 'Sydney tribes' of private school boys dominating the law.

For Simon, the fast pace of the city, pressures of work, physical distance from his parents and a lack of community values in the urban corporate environment militated against appropriate perspective on life. He missed the 'spirituality' of his country home, by which he meant not only its peace and quiet but 'the health of your conscience, I think, and that just means dealing with a lot of issues that you may have; so bereavements, relationships, work and some method of dealing with those things'.

But it was in relation to his family that Simon departed most strikingly from the practices of other corporate men. He and his wife have two young children and he took three months off work when each was born. With the arrival of his second child, both parents chose to work four rather than five days a week in order to share the child-rearing more evenly. 'I see it as much my role as my wife's role,' he said. Despite being in the top 1 per cent of earners nationally, he declared that 'the most important thing to me is my family'.

Simon felt that his career had suffered because of his commitment to family life. He was the only man in his peer group who worked a four-day week, which was unheard of in a senior position. He thought that as a consequence he had been overlooked for a promotion. He was particularly irked by the fact that his boss was a woman who had commented: 'I didn't think you would be interested with your family and your other priorities'. Simon was told that his 'unwillingness to go anywhere at the drop of a hat' was a major reason that he was passed over.

'One of the most difficult aspects,' Simon commented, 'is balancing my own needs from a career point of view versus my family role.' Indeed, he continued to harbour career ambitions even though he wasn't enjoying his job. He was looking for other posts, but had discounted them because of the excess travel. 'I just wonder if it is all worth it,' he mused. 'Maybe there is another way or strategy, so perhaps that is what I am quietly looking for.' He had not yet found it. He was considering giving up a career path to spend even more time at home, but worried about the economic costs: 'I have to educate the kids, you know.'

Patterns of connection

The emotional wellbeing of men is dependent on the quality of their human relationships. However, men commonly have less well-developed social networks than women. The legacy of men's commitment to competition is social isolation. Men then become dependent upon women for their emotional security, a process we are psychologically conditioned for in female-centred childhoods.

Men's reliance on women for emotional sanctuary often does not provide them with the safety they crave. In the modern Western world, women are less dependent on men for their economic survival and less willing to tolerate what they find unacceptable in relationships. This includes the alcohol abuse, infidelity and violence that some men use to disguise the very emotional insecurities they look to women to solve. Men whose self-validation provides security are best able to form successful relationships with others.

Changing social conditions suggest that a new democratisation of personal relationships may now be possible. Men are increasingly aware of the requirement on them to engage in emotional democracy and a few are actively pursuing this ideal. Others are steadfastly resisting it. Most accept the need for more open and negotiated relationships, but are not fully committed through action. One reason for this is the paramount value of work in men's worlds. But since this investment does not provide the emotional connection men need, they turn once more to women – who may no longer be there.

Fortuitously, there are alternatives to paid work or emotional reliance on women for us to connect with others and develop emotional stability. We shall explore some of these strategies in our final two chapters. In chapter 10, we consider the light that Western psychology casts on the stories of desperate men seeking to change their lives towards happiness.

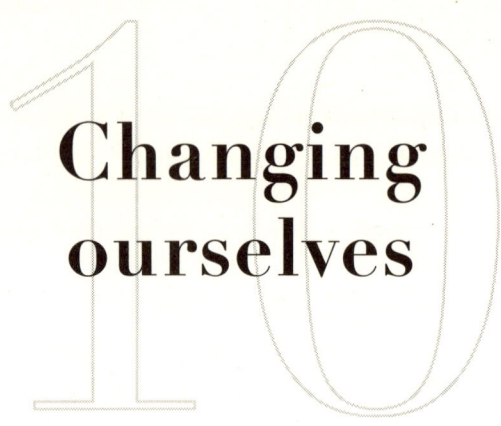

Changing ourselves

Flowing through the pages of this book is a stream of stories centred on depression and unhappy families. In that context, young heroin users and traumatised soldiers received considerable attention. However, a contrasting tributary told of more contented lives, including those of active sportsmen and accepting Diggers. In this chapter, I want to investigate how men can move from discontent to happiness. In particular, we will explore stories about personal change with reference to Western psychology.

We begin with the struggle of young drug users to turn their lives around. The young men from the drop-in centre often expressed a desire to change their drug and crime oriented lifestyle. Most had tried unsuccessfully, but a few showed that it was possible.

Changing lifestyle

A sense of abandonment haunts the emotional lives of drug users, giving rise to anger, anxiety and depression. These men have difficulty trusting other people and struggle with loneliness. For some, despair has cut away their sense of a future and with it any hope of change for the better.

> I don't really think about the future, I don't really have no plans, no goals, nothing. I just think about now and what I'm gonna do today and what I'm gonna do tomorrow; stuff like that. I don't set no goals for the future. (Dane, aged 21)

But all is not lost. Though drugs and alcohol may temporarily ameliorate unpleasant feelings, their long-term use generates new troubles, which paradoxically can prompt men to change their lives. For example, in chapter 4 we met Marcus, who told us: 'The future scares the shit out of me ... Really, I should be looking at myself and where I'm gonna end up ... I know where I'd like to end up with just a normal family, bringing up your daughter or son' (Marcus, aged 20). Marcus points to possibilities of hope and change. The majority of these young men dreamed of futures involving jobs, homes, cars, partners and children; in fact, the whole conventional image of happy family life. Despite their addictions, and because of their past, they hankered after a vision of the 'normal'. On a good day, this dream motivates them to make changes, but they need support to succeed.

DAMIEN'S NEED FOR CHANGE

The young men often told me that they were simply 'fed up with the whole drug lifestyle'.

> I'd had enough of the life. I'd be out of jail for two months and then I'd go back in and I'd miss all my family. I missed my nephew being born. I had no photo of my nephew. I got out and he was four months old and I still hadn't even seen him yet. I'd had enough of my lifestyle; I had to change. If I didn't change, I wouldn't have made it to say, 26. I realised that I had fucked my life up. (Damien, aged 25)

The criminal activity required to fund his drug habit was a particularly problematic aspect of Damien's life.

> I used to be into heaps and heaps of crime, actually. I used to do all that shit, but I got over it; I got sick of it. I'm getting caught now for all the

things that I did ages ago, like I never used to get caught. So that's when I thought give it up now and then in a couple of years time I won't be locked up, you know. I'll get to be free. (Damien, aged 25)

Committing crime troubled a number of the young men ethically. They were not callous criminals but distressed young men doing what was accepted within their cultural milieu. Many were aware of the morally disturbing character of what they were doing and of the possible consequences for their future.

> I haven't stolen for at least seven months. I've just snapped out of that. I just don't want to do crime anymore. I used to break into shops, but I've never broken into someone's house because I feel too guilty doing that. I need the money, but I've got a record now and I don't want a large record 'cause it will affect me when I'm older and looking for a job and I want to get a job eventually and settle down. (Damien, aged 25)

It is not always a lot of fun being homeless and jobless. Certainly, some of the young men enjoyed having the time to hang out and party with mates. However, the attraction of this lifestyle wears off. Sleeping rough and then being moved on by the police takes its toll.

> I lived on the streets for at least six months at the library car park. I used to squat in there; down the bottom of the car park there's a grill you can pull off. Now they have bolted them on so nobody can get in there. I squatted there for at least six, seven months. It's pretty good, but it's not the same as having a roof over your head. I got busted coming out of there one day by Security. I had a bed in there, like I had a mattress in there. I had a stereo. I had candles set up everywhere. I had a table and chairs. They made me clean it all out. I had to run around and find another place to stay; looking for abandoned houses, warehouses, things like that; just running around and wondering where I was going to be each night. (Damien, aged 25)

Damien and his friends also faced the challenge of a growing tolerance to heroin, whereby the initial high gives way to simply avoiding withdrawal symptoms. But quitting isn't easy either; it can be painful, isolating and depressing. The problems of being homeless and jobless do not disappear and daily life is tough without painkilling drugs. And so one quits and falls back, summons up the will to quit again, only to take another tumble, until: 'eventually I just got sick of it and I picked up the phone and dialled the number' (Damien, aged 25).

SUPPORTS FOR CHANGE

A youth worker from the drop-in centre suggested that the young men would eventually relinquish heroin if they lived long enough. His purpose, he told me, was to keep them alive while constantly giving them support and encouragement to change. The young men praised the drop-in centre as a place where they could talk about their problems, receive advice, have breakfast, take a shower, talk to friends and recover some dignity. The centre operated on a minimal budget in run-down facilities, but provided enormously good value to the community. It is cheaper than prison and offers more hope of reducing crime.

Relationships with girlfriends and children generated the most compelling reasons for these men to transform their lives. A number of them recognised that they were not offering the environment their children needed. Dave was a heroin user for three years, during which time he met a woman and they had a child. After a separation and reconciliation, they were 'together' again, but living separately. She had laid down conditions for cohabitation, which was providing the motivation for him to enter a detox program.

> I have to prove to her that I can stop using first. I've been looking after my daughter when she goes to work. She used to leave her with her mum, but now I do it because I want to get trusted. So I'll stop using. This way I can prove to her that I'm not using. She wrote it down on a piece of paper and I had to sign it. I have to give her money towards the baby; money for herself and to pay the bills and to stop using and I had to sign it. (Dave, aged 23)

Of course, if girlfriends were also drug users, the partnership could hinder rather than promote recovery. However, for Marcus and Jane a moment arrived when they said to themselves: 'We gotta do it for the kids, the kids come first no matter what.' Jane's mother, who had previously banned them from her house, responded positively to their willingness and agreed to act as their 'carer' in the aftermath of a residential detox program. Right now, Marcus and his partner are clean, but then this was their third attempt.

The motivation for these men to change their lives was a combination of hope and despair. They were 'pushed' out of their routines by homelessness, crime, the police, jail, and a general weariness with the drug lifestyle. They were 'pulled' towards happiness by girlfriends, children and hopes for a more stable future. Most of the young men were at least contemplating the need for change. Indeed, the majority had gone beyond contemplation to action, having been through a detox program, or quit alone. Nonetheless, since most had also returned to old ways, it is worth considering the general principles of self-change, and the experiences of men who have achieved longer-term success.

Emotion and the process of change

WHAT WE NEED TO CHANGE

There are things we can change and things we can't. For example, we can't alter a genetic inheritance towards 'sensitivity'. However, reconstructing the way we think can reduce its capacity for suffering and maximise its creative potential. As we learn to interpret our world, we build up personal maps of meaning that make sense of life and guide us through it. Thinking is at the core of our emotions; it is not events that make us happy or miserable, but our interpretation of them. Since it is our stories that make us happy or lead us to despair, so it is our stories that we need to change. We can learn to observe, describe and amend our thoughts and thus our emotions.

We met Stephen on the first page of this book. Since infancy, he had constructed a story-world filled with fear, loss and abandonment. He had experienced a chaotic family life with an alcoholic father who resorted to violence. Stephen's mother fled with her child into a life of single-parenthood blighted by poverty. By contrast, we also met Harold whose parents had separated as well, but who continued to feel loved by them. He was able to develop a more constructive and positive outlook.

We know of at least two consequences that flow from Stephen's insecure childhood: first, changes in his brain strengthen his fearful responses; and second, he constructs a blame-saturated story in which he is never 'good enough'. Harold, however, was able to develop a self-story involving acceptance of his shortcomings. He had constructed a mental map in which his life had a purpose and worth. His brain chemistry enabled him to experience joy in his work and achievements.

The biochemistry of the brain and the stories we tell ourselves are two sides of the same coin. As we construct one, we constitute the other; when we change one, we change the other. If we take drugs, we change the way we think (and so antidepressants have their use), but we can also change our biochemistry by altering our thoughts (hence the value of cognitive therapy). Emotion can be understood as a matrix of interacting elements, including our conscious thought processes, brain biochemistry (of which we are not self-aware), the physiology of the body (heart racing, pupil dilation, and so on), and cultural-linguistic interpretations.

The matrix of emotion

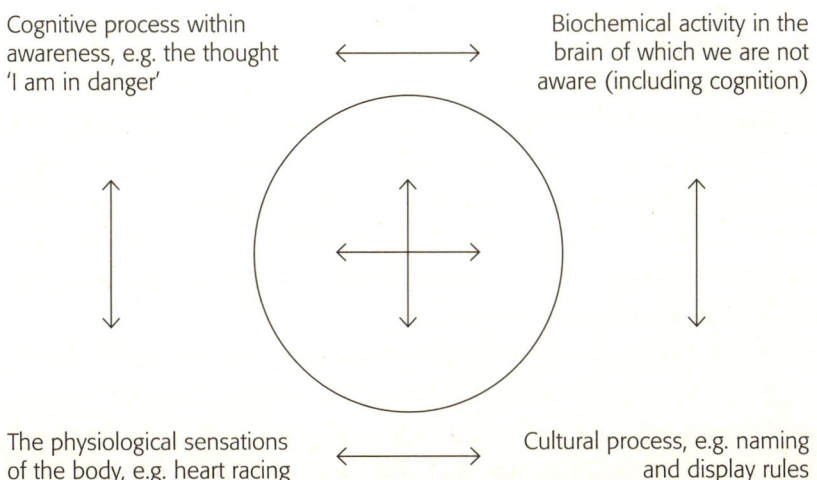

HOW WE CAN CHANGE

We can move our mental constructs away from despair and towards happiness. Therapy makes us aware of the stories that we tell ourselves, enabling us to change them. Just as we seek to understand ourselves by telling stories, so we can adopt new ones that improve our wellbeing. We can reinterpret the past in ways that offer joy in the present moment and hope for the future. For example, I once told myself an angry story about a drunken and irrational father who caused me suffering. I now tell myself a narrative of reconciliation about a man who suffered a lot in which no one is to blame.

To change ourselves, we must enter a reinforcing spiral by which shifting thoughts improve our emotions, and thus our behaviour, and thus our thoughts, and thus our emotions, and so forth. The portal of this spiral of change could be behaviour or body–brain biochemistry (for example, exercise or medication). However, because cognitive processes are at the core of emotions, much therapeutic work focuses on thinking. Being mindful of our thoughts enables us to rewrite the narrative of our lives and amend our neural pathways.

A spiral of change

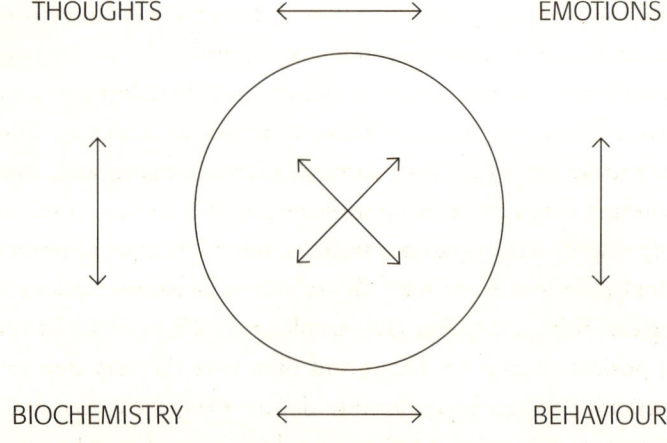

'Reframing' is a significant self-change skill that we can learn by which we innovatively redescribe our experience; that is, we put a new frame or story around it. Instead of thinking of past troubles as lifelong burdens, we can think of them as gifts that teach us better ways to live (see Frank's story in chapter 11). Rather than blame our parents for the things we think they did to us, we can understand that if they could have acted differently they would have. And instead of thinking that we are a social 'failure' because we don't have 25 friends, we can revel in the one we do have. In short, we water the seeds of happiness rather than those of misery.

Nonetheless, it is hard to tell hopeful stories if we are already filled with fear, anxiety and sadness. First, we need to calm the mind and regulate our emotions. Psychologist Marsha Lineham[1] offers us a set of useful techniques to achieve this that combine cognitive behaviour therapy with mindfulness meditation (see chapter 11).

We begin by more skilfully identifying our emotions through observing and describing events, which includes our interpretation of them. She suggests that we *keep an emotion dairy* that records events, interpretations, bodily feelings and action urges. We thereby increase our mindfulness to current emotions, and experience them without judging or inhibiting them. We are asked to *observe our emotion*, note its presence – and step back. The key is to accept our emotion rather than push it away, because this simply adds an extra layer of suffering. Remember, you are not your emotion, says Lineham, and you need not act on it.

Lineham then encourages us to reduce our vulnerability to 'emotion mind' by avoiding stress that increases emotional reactivity. She first urges us to *take care of the body* through exercise, eating well, avoiding mood-altering drugs and getting sufficient sleep. Lineham is not asking us simply to attend to unpleasant feelings, but to generate pleasant ones. Accordingly, we seek to *increase the number of pleasurable events* in life by doing one thing a day that gives us pleasure. We can start by making a list of positive events we desire; and then take the first step towards it. In particular, we are encouraged to do one thing a day that makes us feel competent and we are urged to attend to our relationships since our connections to others are vital to our wellbeing.

When we feel destructively self-critical, we are encouraged to *take opposite action*, giving ourself a sense of mastery. If you feel fear, do a little of what you are afraid of. In the face of sadness and lethargy, get active; and when you feel angry, imagine sympathy towards another, and act on it. Lineham asks us to *tolerate negative emotions* without taking impulsive action. She offers us a number of ways to live with emotional distress, including:

- *Distract* yourself with positive activities such as hobbies or visiting a friend.
- *Self-soothe* the five senses: buy a flower, listen to beautiful music, have a good meal.
- *Improve the moment* through meditation or relaxing the body.
- *Encourage yourself* by saying 'I can do it'; or 'It will pass'.
- *Calm the mind* by learning to follow the breath and put a half-smile on the face.
- *Develop radical acceptance* by deciding to accept reality – let yourself go into 'what is'.

Stories of change

Research psychologists James Prochaska, John Norcross and Carlo DeClementi[2] have identified a series of steps included in many stories of personal change. Their model does not map neatly onto everyone's experience, but it does act as a guide to the processes; starting with the truism that in order to change one must want to change.

Our quest for change begins by thinking about our need for it; for example, we may, like Marcus, come to feel that we simply cannot continue as we are (*contemplation stage*). After a while, we develop more determination and develop a strategy to do so (*decision stage*). For example, Marcus and Jane (see chapter 7) decided to stop using drugs and made a plan to enter a detox unit, supported by Jane's mother. The next step is to put the plan into action; for example, Marcus and Jane successfully quit heroin with the help of a residential program (*action stage*). However, change is a process that needs to be continuously supported (*maintenance stage*). No doubt, Marcus and Jane would benefit from the activities suggested by Lineham. Not all of the young men from the drop-in centre wanted to change, and many of those that did were unable to maintain it. However, Daniel and Patrick demonstrate that it can be done.

DANIEL'S STORY

Daniel (aged 35) is the son of English middle-class parents. He left school and home at 16 to work on the docks. At 20, he was serving a year in jail for possessing and dealing in heroin. On completion of his sentence, and after a short delay thinking through his life, Daniel returned to education, working his way towards a PhD and employment as a university researcher.

Daniel told me that as a young man he lacked self-confidence, attributing this to his father, who was a 'control freak' and 'a bit too anal for my liking'. As a consequence of his dad 'always telling me what to do and how to do it', he felt that he didn't gain the life skills that enable self-assurance. He attributed his drug addiction to anxiety and specifically to his fear of failure. Like the young men from the drop-in centre, Daniel points to the painkilling properties of drugs as their central attraction:

> What the heroin crowd share in common is the inability to handle and organise their life in a way that fulfils them; instead of making the effort, they have just chosen to use the drugs as an anaesthetic … Too scared to fail I think was one of my problems. I didn't want to try because I was worried about failure, probably my father being such an oppressive guy and he was a model for me that sort of freaked me out a bit, I don't know why. So I didn't want to fail maybe for that reason. (Daniel, aged 35)

It is a truism of the therapeutic literature that addicts must want to stop before they can succeed. Daniel is not unusual (see Patrick below) in getting to a point where he felt life could not get much worse.

> So the thing that really used to freak me out and make me depressed was looking at life and thinking 'Well, there it is, but I don't dare try and

> grab it' and so the change I guess was just getting so low that I thought it can't be that bad, just get out and give it a go and see what you think. (Daniel, aged 35)

Personal change for Daniel involved a shift of 'mindset'; that is, transforming the set of personal constructs or thought patterns that made up his world. In particular, he needed to face his fear of failure and take more control of his life.

> And I kind of rediscovered what I think I'd found when I was really young, that things were really quite easy, that I could do a lot of things that I saw other people do. I didn't have to be scared and I think it was just the scared aspect that was making me see everything so negatively. I had that kind of mindset and I think the change was just getting so low that I thought I didn't know the way to go so I might as well just try this and it can't get any worse. So I tried it and I kept going. (Daniel, aged 35)

Overcoming a heroin addiction requires a complete change in lifestyle, since 'one of the best ways to get yourself off it is to just leave all your old habits and your friends behind'. You have to leave behind not just the drug, but the whole social world that supports it. Prison seems to have played a significant role in this for Daniel. Quite apart from the fact that 'only a madman shoots up in prison', it gave him time to 'just sit down and think and try and work out what was wrong and what I had to do to sort it out'. He learnt to talk more positively to himself, so that 'it will start off negative and then eventually I'll think that's good and that's good and that's good'.

Daniel felt the need for control over his life in order to give him confidence and self-respect: a strategy similar to that of his father, whose achievements he admires but whose authority he tried to escape. Yet, he came to recognise that some of the 'anal qualities' of his father that he disliked could be the basis for his own achievements. 'It's interesting how the negative influences in your life can end up being quite positive,' he said. So on release from prison Daniel adopted the 'rigid disciplined approach' required for the public achievement that would impress his dad and himself.

Daniel was to find pleasure and purpose in the process of getting a doctorate and learning to play music. In particular, he found a new way to think about himself through mastering new skills that gave his life a sense of purpose. Daniel's change of lifestyle gave him a sense of competence in and over himself. He developed skills of self-discipline that gave him confidence in his own solidity and greater assurance in the world.

Like many men, including his father the 'control freak', Daniel hoped then that external validation would give his life meaning, and it certainly helped. However, on gaining his doctorate, 'it failed to impress me'. Though he had still not quite overcome his sense of being 'not good enough', Daniel was able to tell a story about relinquishing heroin through self-discipline and 'changing his mind'.

PATRICK'S STORY

Patrick was 26 when I met him. He had been a heavy drinker and marijuana smoker from his early teens. At 17, he became a heroin addict and remained so for five years. When I spoke to him, he had been free of drug addiction for four years; he no longer used heroin or any illegal drugs, nor did he drink alcohol. Our conversation centred on the background to his addiction and the pathways he took towards recovery. This was not an easy route for him; it took courage and determination.

As a young man, Patrick felt considerable anger towards his alcoholic father for his emotional 'absence'. They argued at lot, which Patrick attributes to his father's authoritarianism and his own 'deep anger'. He grew up feeing close to his mother, but also felt somewhat smothered by her. Patrick wondered if she had sought from him the emotional and physical support lacking in her husband. He recounted the frequent parental arguments he witnessed and his own subsequent guilt. Patrick also told me of the anger he felt towards his mother for tolerating his father's threatening behaviour. He explained that as a child he had been the subject of sexual abuse from an older man, but he did not elaborate.

Patrick had found the exploration of father–son relationships by men's movement writers like Steve Biddulph and John Lee valuable to him. He told me that he and many other male addicts had difficult relationships with their fathers, suggesting that they search for a 'high' in order to cover over the 'father–son wound': 'We put drugs in that wound, in the hole to make us feel good, to kind of fill us up.'

> I look back now and I wasn't aware of it at the time but I fitted in with brokenness, with broken people; people with a similar childhood and I kind of had that connection with those people. We used drugs together and we just did things together. I guess heroin was to wipe the world out. I didn't have to feel anything. I didn't have to be responsible for anything. It was easy to continue to blame the world. I guess when I wasn't on drugs I was very angry, impatient, intolerant.
>
> That's the kind of person I was. When I was on drugs I had the sense of a euphoric feeling; the sense that I'm okay, I feel good; an extra kind of high; an extra lift. Not only did I feel that euphoric feeling, I felt superior. I was superman flying without a cape. I was bulletproof. (Patrick, aged 26)

To finance his drug habit, Patrick undertook criminal activities that eventually led to a year in jail, during which time his second child was born. This was a particularly poignant moment for him as his own father had been in prison the day that he was born. This realisation prompted a number of attempts to give up drugs, which were unsuccessful because of 'the simple fact that I wasn't ready to change my whole lifestyle'. But this was to be transformed:

> My sister had died six months before of a heroin overdose and there were people just dropping left, right and centre. Old friends were doing big jail sentences. I just knew I would be the next to die or I would be the next to get a jail sentence, because many nights I would go around robbing a garage or something like that. I guess the spiritual bankruptcy. I felt the meaningless and monotonous life I had. I wanted some meaning to life, so I went to detox; it was shocking. I wanted to have a girlfriend. I wanted to change my life and I really wanted it and I was willing to make a sacrifice. (Patrick, aged 26)

The reasons Patrick offers to explain his triumph over addiction revisit some familiar themes: weariness with the lifestyle, the threat of jail, the very real possibility of death and the lack of meaning or spiritual purpose (see chapter 7). One night, he sat alone in a toilet preparing to shoot up. In his mind he saw himself sitting there, needle in hand. He felt fatigued by his life, seeing only the pointlessness of his existence; he squirted the heroin down the bowl. This was to prove a crucial turning point: 'This time when I got clean I realised that nothing in my life was healthy and that I had to change everything; absolutely every part of my life.'

Patrick's determination to change his life was a significant reason for his success, but he still needed the right enabling conditions. His aunt's (a psychologist) willingness to house and support him throughout his detox and the subsequent year was vital; as was the care his ex-partner showed in taking him to Narcotics Anonymous (NA), where he met people he fitted in with to support his recovery. By staying with his aunt, Patrick moved far from his circle of drug-using friends; and by entering NA he was able to make new ones. Finally, he undertook a process of therapy that enabled him to understand better the source of his addictions in neediness and emotional pain.

It was a crucial part of Patrick's successful recovery that, unlike the many continuing addicts to whom I spoke, he learnt to master a language of emotional growth: 'I had to go back to learn how to feel because I didn't know how to feel.' He found therapy a useful way to explore addictions that sprung from his attempts to 'medicate this wound inside'. And he engaged with the language of Christian 'spirituality', which he told me was 'probably the most important thing for me'.

> I believe in God and I need to commit, have belief and have faith in something greater than me. Not only did my friends in NA help me get clean, but I believe today God has a purpose for me. I'm just aware of what my will is and what God's will is for me and I have that awareness on a daily basis. God wants me to be open to growing all the time. He wants me to be alive. (Patrick, aged 26)

Patrick's mother had given him a Catholic upbringing, but he had been unable to accept it. Indeed, while he had a vague belief in the divine as a young man, he was also angry with God. However, his auntie, Narcotics Anonymous and a friendship with a Christian woman helped to change his mind. He now felt that the counselling work he was doing with a drug agency and the pursuit of appropriate therapeutic activities was God's plan for him. Patrick had found a sense of purpose in his life and a language with which to speak it that was vital to his wellbeing (see chapter 11).

Between them, Daniel and Patrick demonstrate the critical components of any strategy for self-change, especially overcoming addiction. First and foremost, one must want to change, a desire that is often prompted by a sense that 'things couldn't get worse'. It is then important to attend to patterns of thinking that support damaging habits in order to transform them; for example, the thought that one is 'not good enough'. For addicts, it is usually necessary to leave behind their social world and construct a new one. Any personal transformation also requires self-discipline and the acquisition of an appropriate language of emotion. Above all, successful self-change requires a new sense of purpose in life, whether this is through study like Daniel, or in spirituality like Patrick.

Men's groups: Working on yourself

Daniel and Patrick participate in a society increasingly saturated with talk about self-development. The psychological professions now act as a modern priesthood, explaining to us how we 'work' and how best we can be 'fixed'. Psychology has not remained within the university nor stayed on the couch, but rather appears as a force within popular culture through the proliferation of self-help media. Popular psychology is now a powerful stream of thought in contemporary culture that shapes our behaviour and identities.

Across the media spectrum, we are the targets of psychologically motivated advice about how best to conduct our emotional selves (including in this book). For every psychological or behavioural difficulty there is a book, a TV show, a website and self-help group. This exhortation to personal development can fuel a self-absorbed obsession with our own problems, displacing thoughts for others. However, Western psychology also offers genuinely skilful means to forge constructive change. Indeed, a consistent theme of my conversations with 'men's movement' activists was the idea of 'working on oneself'.

BRUCE AND COLIN TALK EMOTION

Bruce paused to reflect on what he had been saying:

> I hope I have given you the impression that I've been working on my stuff, to use that wonderful psychological expression, in order to clear myself of expectations and judgments and purely being the victim of my story. I had to get rid of a whole load of expectations that I just brought out of my life and dumped them on whoever was my partner. I have struggled not to be in my stuff, not to be in my assumptions or expectations; not to be in judgment about the way I should be or other people should be. (Bruce, aged 54)

Bruce repeatedly applied the phrase 'unconscious man' to himself and his father; he described the process of 'becoming conscious' through 'working on oneself' as being 'mindful'. Indeed, participants in 'men's groups' understood themselves to be undertaking a process of self-aware transformation. As Colin told me:

> I have wasted a lot of time in trying to get to know other people when getting to know me is a more meaningful, powerful, real thing. I can change me, I can't change other people and if I change me and how I am in the world, I see that things are different for me, around me. It changes my relationships and people generally respond to that. (Colin, aged 48)

For Colin, emotions are the usual target of self-improvement because he felt men struggle to articulate their feelings. He suggested that the work of men's groups is to undo that conditioning. 'Most of the issues that bring men into men's groups stem from their emotions,' he added. 'One of the biggest problems for men is their poor ability to express emotions because they are proud and hold too much in.'

However, it is the public requirement not to show vulnerability that underpins men's reluctance to express emotion rather than an inability to do so, suggested Richard (aged 46). Men do experience emotions and can express them, he said, but difficulties arise from uncertainty surrounding which feelings they can express, under what circumstances and how this should be done. He pointed out that men frequently express anger but do not always articulate love, especially in ways women expect. For Richard, men's groups provide a forum for exploring relationships and the cultural rules of emotion. Other men have turned to spiritual teachers (see chapter 11) or to the growing literature on happiness.

The positive psychology of happiness

Martin Seligman[3] is the pivotal figure in what he calls the 'positive psychology' of happiness. He suggests that happiness, joy and love are rooted in our evolutionary need for solidarity, while 'looking after number one' promotes only sadness. Sociability and human relationships, then, have supported our survival and development. Though we are temperamentally predisposed to be more or less happy (or depressed), Seligman thinks that we can nevertheless increase contentment in our lives.

Modern minds may be surprised to learn that the accumulation of wealth does *not* appear crucial to happiness. After reviewing an array of evidence, Seligman concludes that although wealth is initially connected to life satisfaction, once a nation reaches an annual gross domestic product of US$8000 per capita the correlation between wealth and life satisfaction disappears. He suggests that the importance we place on money is more significant in determining happiness than the amount of money we actually have. In particular, our perception of how much wealth we possess in relation to other people matters more than the total amounts of money involved. People who value money more than other goals are less satisfied with their incomes and their lives. What we think about money generally counts for more than our objective circumstances.

Seligman's exploration of correlations between happiness and marriage, social life, health, education, climate, race, gender and religion generates a mixed picture. Marriage is positively correlated with greater levels of life satisfaction, but the causality is not clear. Marriage may make us happier, but then again maybe happier people get married more – and stay married longer. Education, climate, race and gender are not strongly connected to levels of happiness. Religion is associated with life satisfaction, probably because it promotes sociability, optimism, hope and a sense of purpose.

A PATH TO HAPPINESS

Seligman's most reliable conclusions are that the richer one's social world and the greater one's optimism, the happier one is. Our happiness is built through connections to other people rather than through individual achievement and depends more on our patterns of thinking than upon actual events. He suggests that to promote greater happiness we should foster forgiveness and gratitude about the past, savour the present moment, and look to the future with hope and optimism.

Seligman's prescriptions for the past and future are cognitive in orientation. They entail deliberately cultivating particular ways of thinking. For example, rather than ruminating on the slights of the past, contentment comes through being grateful for that which went well and developing forgiveness towards people who caused us suffering. We can encourage this outlook by writing a 'Gratitude Diary' in which we record the things in life we are grateful for. In this way, we extend 'good' memories and downplay the 'bad' ones.

Cultivating optimism and hope generates happiness. To do so, Seligman recommends that we pay attention to the characteristic way that we think about events. For the pessimist, 'bad events' are held to be personal, pervasive and permanent. For example, a poor test result is interpreted as a disaster for my whole life and a consequence of inherent stupidity. By contrast, optimists see difficulties as temporary, domain-specific and external in their origination. Here my exam marks are understood as merely a passing setback that occurred because it was so hot that day, and anyway they will have little bearing on the most important things in life. Hope stems from finding permanent and universal explanations for 'positive events' but temporary and specific causes for the negative ones.

We can build up the optimism upon which happiness depends by monitoring our thinking and challenging negative interpretations of events, suggests Seligman. He urges us to explore the evidence for our negative thoughts and to dispute them by considering less singular explanations for troubles. For example, if at first we think that our test results will ruin our life, we need to stop and explore these beliefs for their veracity. Beliefs are not facts; aren't there other paths we could take? Couldn't we retake the test and do better next time? Aren't there lots of occasions in which we have overcome adversity?

Seligman recommends that we cultivate the condition of 'flow' in the present moment, by which one is so absorbed in activity that time stops. Flow emerges through concentration on a challenging task that requires a degree of skill we can meet, but not too easily. This gives us a sense of control and effortless involvement whereby the self vanishes. Flow is a side effect of worthwhile action rather than the overt pursuit of pleasure. It appears when one is taken 'outside' of the self, whereas self-absorption is a feature of depression. I find that a state of flow can be achieved through writing, while for others playing sport or music might be the favoured route.

As we shall see in chapter 11, paying attention to our thoughts and self-consciously developing gratitude is also a feature of mindfulness meditation. Seligman certainly concurs with an emphasis on positive engagement with the present moment. There is also considerable agreement between Eastern and Western psychology about the connection between health, happiness and ethics.

COMMUNITY, ETHICS AND HAPPINESS

Seligman proposes that our deepest emotional satisfactions come through the exercise of strengths and virtues (gratifications) rather than from the pursuit of pleasure. He suggests that, rather than asking 'How can I be happy?', we should instead ask 'What is the good life?' He defines *the good life* as 'using one's signature strengths to obtain abundant gratification in the main realms of your life'.[4] Signature strengths are personal psychological characteristics and skills with a moral dimension, such as curiosity and the pursuit of knowledge, or integrity and the value of justice (Seligman lists 24 such strengths).

Happiness, then, involves the pursuit of 'right action' or virtue. Here ethics only make sense in the context of a whole way of life or culture that defines the 'good'. Hence, happiness depends not just on 'the good life' but also on *the meaningful life*, which involves 'using your signature strengths and virtues in the service of something much larger than you are'.[5]

Western psychologists know that isolation breeds depression and note that 'failure to thrive' in children derives from lack of attention and weak attachment to others. In this way, they connect happiness to healthy human relationships. Nevertheless, Western psychology does tend to focus on the individual. By contrast, Eastern thinking places notions of community and interconnection or 'interbeing'[6] at the core of its teachings and practice. Our happiness is dependent on the happiness of others. It is thus in our interests to reduce all forms of suffering. This stress on interconnection encourages ethical behaviour and the development of compassion. Our personal happiness is built on the pursuit of virtue and the reduction of suffering for all. In the next chapter, we explore in more detail Western men who have looked to spiritual teachings for inspiration and the meaningful life.

Redemption song

We all hope for a happy, peaceful and meaningful life. As psychologists Danah Zohar and Ian Marshall suggest, we share 'a specifically human longing to find meaning and value in what we do and experience ... We have a longing for something that gives us and our actions a sense of worth'.[1] For us to find value in our life depends on viewing it in a wider meaning-giving context; whether this is our family, our friends, a political commitment, a football club, our work, our religious framework or the cosmos itself. A happy life is a meaningful life and a meaningful life is one in which we have purpose. Purpose entails a relationship to something more expansive than us.

In this chapter, we will investigate men who are committed to developing emotional wellbeing through the 'spiritual' practices of mindfulness and meditation. These activities are part of an Eastern psychology of contentment. Indeed, the Western psychology of happiness we encountered in chapter 10 has drawn extensively from these traditions. The word 'spiritual' as I use it in this chapter has nothing to do with a supernatural deity or a 'thing' called spirit. Rather, it is a signpost pointing to practices of self-conscious awareness and contemplation. It is part of the search for peace, meaning and happiness.

DAVID: DEVELOPING AN INNER STRENGTH

David was an Anglo-Australian and former Thai-based Buddhist monk. He told me that his experience of spiritual life had been a direct challenge to core Western notions of masculinity.

> Whilst I am now a lay person and am involved in the things lay people do, finding my spirituality allows me to have a perspective on my experience of being alive as a human being, as a man. Here are men living in many ways a way of life that many people would say isn't masculine. They're not exerting their masculinity through their language, through the clothes they wear, through their behaviours, through involvement with women; and yet there was something about them, something that was deep and strong. It was like a spiritual strength that was there. I found that inspiring. (David, aged 37)

David felt that his monastic experience offered him a perspective on masculinity that departed from the ascendant Western view. Monks are, of course, expressing a particular style of manhood through their language, clothes and actions. However, David is suggesting that the ways of monks are more desirable than those of conventional modern men. The gentleness of language and behaviour characteristic of Thai monks is contrasted to the implied aggression of Westerners. Likewise, while the clothing of monks is deliberately plain, so that of Western men is for display. The monks are described as 'deep and strong' so that, by implication, Western masculinity is deemed somewhat superficial.

The idea of strength is a core characteristic of conventional Western notions about men. However, it is recast here to suggest not physical but mental and emotional potency. Spiritual practices often contain notions of endurance and acceptance that are also characteristic of our pre-1960s male conventions (for example, the Diggers). While David is declining Western masculinity, he is simultaneously redescribing and reclaiming one of its core characteristics; that is, the idea of personal 'inner' depth and power. His contention chimes with Susan Faludi's case that an 'ornamental culture' of celebrity, image, entertainment and marketing has turned masculinity into a matter of display rather than celebrating personal qualities of character, confidence and purpose (see chapter 3).

David's father displayed qualities similar to those of the monks he admired. Although as a child his father 'was a bit of an embarrassment' to him, being quite different from other local fathers, David thought him wise: 'I looked up to him and respected him.' His father was stoical in the face of a life-threatening medical condition and encouraged David's family to 'live a fairly simple life'. For example, they did not have a television set.

> His attitudes and thriftiness, carefulness, became very much a part of our growing up as well. We respected nature; we respected life, animal life, but also we were careful how we spent our money and really looked after things as well as we could. I'd say my parents, especially my father, was quite a strict parent and so that instilled within me a respect for the law, a respect for, a sense of morality, a sense of self-discipline as well. (David, aged 37)

David's father was attracted to Buddhism and took his son to the local temple, where David 'felt a connectedness to the monks; quiet, calm, serene people, men'. Throughout David's childhood, his father modelled the values of independence, self-sufficiency, thriftiness, carefulness, stoicism, respect for life, morality and self-discipline to him. Later, in a Thai monastery where 'it was austere but there was a sense of joy that came from living very simply', David was to find those values again. Courtesy of globalisation, David connects the pre-modern discourses of Buddhism to his father's 1950s values. In doing so, he critiques the ornamental masculinity of contemporary culture. That is, character virtues such as strength of mind and care for others are contrasted with the superficiality of consumer exhibition.

It is often said that David's father's generation lacked emotional intelligence. However, David thought his father 'more emotionally aware than my mother; more emotionally sensitive in a good way and yet, you know, he was always a very masculine man ... I felt he was a wise man ... I felt very close to him'. In a Thai monastery, David also found that:

> There was an emotional fulfilment through talking to the other monks and so an emotional intelligence that was there, that I guess was more

real and emotional than what men tend to think is emotional life, which is basically just physical, sexual life. (David, aged 37)

A problem of our time

If we compare David to Marcus (see chapter 4), Toby (see chapter 7), or any of the more troubled men who populate the pages of this book, he looks like an exceptional and fortunate man. He has been able to cultivate a meaningful and emotionally balanced life. Yet, we live in times when our culture poses particular obstacles to achieving this condition. The people of pre-modern societies had living traditions of family, community, morality and Gods into which they were embedded and which endowed them with purpose. Modern Western societies have fewer such meaningful collective traditions or communities. The conventional family is in disarray and our God has been declared well and truly dead. We live in atomised societies where the central institutions are geared to individuals rather than to communities.

Our day-to-day lives are largely cut off from direct experience of sickness, madness, criminality, sexuality and death that would raise vital existential and moral questions.[2] The sick and dying are segregated from us in hospitals, enabling us to forget that it is in our nature to grow old, to get sick and to die. In cultures where death is more visible, it is made meaningful through ritual stories that give life its sacred character. In Western cultures, we hide away much that is intrinsic to life but which might threaten our emotional security, including death and mental illness. Our culture then struggles to provide us with the answers to life's 'big' questions that are necessary to a full and satisfying existence.

Ironically, as we have sought to reduce our fear of death and sickness through material 'progress', contemporary culture has generated new forms of anxiety: notably the continual requirement for individual decision-making without reliable maps. Driven by an obsession with 'the economy', we are more concerned with personal consumer choice than with meaningful relationships. We may say we value our families and friends above all things, but our practices say something different. We spend more time working and shopping than belonging within a community. Under those circumstances, we must depend on our individual stories without the guidance of a broader meaningful context. Lacking surety, our life choices become an anxiety-inducing process and meaninglessness a fundamental problem of our time.

DISEASES OF MEANING

Men's psychological and cultural training makes us particularly vulnerable to hyper-individualism, which cuts us off from each other and from wider community narratives. We are often more individualistic, success-oriented and competitive than women. We lack the social networks that sustain the human heart (see chapter 9). In that context, we might understand men as suffering from 'diseases of meaning'. Meaning is linked to emotion because the way we think is a vital component of how we feel. The thought that our life lacks purpose, or that we have failed to live up to our ideals, is constitutive of emptiness, anxiety, anger and depression. Contemporary men face change and loss in their relationships with work, women and the family (see chapter 3) without alternative collective value systems to draw on.

Yet, paradoxically, the contemporary stress on individuals making themselves anew also presents us with the opportunity to constructively reshape ourselves. For example, Western culture is now witnessing a resurgence of interest in 'spirituality' that contributes to a meaningful life, but which is distanced from 'organised religion'.[3] The variety of global cultural traditions now available means that we can find new answers to the question of what it is to be a man – or more significantly, the value of being human together.

Mike told me that, during a period of self-fashioning prompted by depression, 'the spirituality came first'. He found meaning in being an at-home father and offering 'service' to others through the men's movement. For Mark, the idea of spirituality was inseparable from emotional development. He pointed to the experience of being 'dispirited' to indicate what it meant to him. Bruce, who organised a men's group, saw spirituality as 'doing anything mindfully. I think that when you are sufficiently mindful you are having a spiritual experience'.

The men's movement sometimes appears to me as unreflective new age mythology or as a reactionary return to traditional 'family values'. However, at its best these men are engaging in mindfulness, emotional communication and the development of a compassionate ethics. They are seeking to remake themselves and their personal relationships in more self-conscious and democratic ways. That said, depression prompted me to explore the benefits of mindfulness meditation rather than the men's movement. In particular, I was attracted to the convergence of Buddhism with psychotherapy. As such, my discussion stages an 'East meets West' dialogue, as befits this era of globalisation.

Eastern psychology meets Western men

The magazine *Psychology Today* (October 2006) suggests that 10 million Americans participate in meditation of some kind. Much of it is underpinned by Eastern psychology. Indeed, spiritual practices are becoming increasingly influential within Western psychology and self-help philosophies. Their attraction lies in a combination of individual growth and a sense of community. The most influential of the Eastern spiritual traditions in the West is Buddhism. This philosophy tells us that we experience discontent or 'unsatisfactory-ness' because we cling to our desires when reality is impermanent and cannot be bent to our will. The solution proposed is a path of meditative practice, mindfulness and ethics leading to self-awareness in the context of community.

MEDITATION AND MINDFULNESS

Meditation entails two key elements: concentration and 'insight'. Buddhist teacher Thich Nhat Hanh calls this 'stopping and calming', which enables 'deep looking'. The practice involves developing the capacity to place attention on one single point. This is commonly the in-and-out movement of the breath. As concentration is strengthened, the mind settles, we become more peaceful, and understanding grows.

To act skilfully in the world and increase our contentment, we need to be mindful of what is happening right now. Mindfulness involves deliberately and purposefully placing one's attention on the present moment in a non-judgmental fashion. When we are walking, we need to be conscious that we are walking. When we are sitting, we need to know that we are sitting.[4]

> ### *Mindfulness of the breath*
> 1. Settle into a comfortable sitting position, keeping your back straight.
> 2. Bring your awareness to the breath as it moves in and out of your body. You can do this either at the entrance to the nostrils or on your lower abdomen.
> 3. When your mind wanders off, as it will, note where it has gone then gently bring it back to the breath.
> 4. Practise this activity for ten minutes a day, building it up to 40 minutes.
> 5. In stressful situations, stop and follow the breath, if only for a couple of minutes.

There are many ways to develop mindfulness in daily life other than sitting on a cushion. Mindfulness is meditation in action. We might pick a routine activity each day and make a special effort to be mindful during it. For example, we might concentrate on mindful eating or cleaning our teeth.

Mindfulness brings our conscious attention to immediate experience without struggling to change it. And if we pay attention to our emotions, we come to appreciate the conditions under which they arise, what they feel like and how best to deal with them. We become less attached to them and more able to make self-conscious choices. Faced with difficult emotions, we might say to ourselves: 'Feelings come and go like clouds in a windy sky. Conscious breathing is my anchor'.[5] We can also set out to cultivate particular states of mind such as compassion or loving-kindness. These are the kinds of practices that engaged the Western men I spoke with.

CHARLES: A SPIRITUAL HOME

Charles described how, at the age of 16, he suffered what he thought was 'some kind of a nervous breakdown' in which:

> I suddenly instantaneously saw that all concepts are just concepts. So of course everything that I thought that I was and everything that I planned to do, all of which I took to be real, suddenly I could see they're not real. It was like God had just disappeared [Charles relinquished his Catholic faith] and I was in this black, utterly alone, total aloneness, and it would be like that forever. And the side effect was depression, like I was deeply depressed for years. (Charles, aged 50)

During Charles's lengthy struggle with depression, he encountered meditation. This prompted sustained study visits to South-East Asia and Hawaii to further his practice.

> My concentration was developing and as the concentration develops the mind calms down and you start to let go of a lot of stuff. So when I meditated I felt really good. And I was doing a lot of meditation in Hawaii. So generally I felt pretty good, unusually so in comparison. It was a paradise in comparison with anything that I had been through since I was 16. (Charles, aged 50)

Meditation enabled Charles to feel better than he did in his more usual state of misery and he deploys a metaphor from his Catholic background, 'paradise', to describe his new condition. Over time, his confidence in Buddhist practices grew until he joined a South-East Asia monastery to live as a monk. He had found his 'spiritual home'. That is:

> A place where you are comfortable and where you can practise the dharma[6] ... a place where you feel that it's natural, that what you are doing is natural and that it belongs in this culture, and it belongs to who you are and where you come from and how you behave as a person. And you've got friends; friendship is really important because if you don't have friends you are in trouble ... a life that isn't based on simply gaining material possessions or position; that goes deeper than that. That to me is a spiritual life. But because of the mental suffering that I've been through and the suffering that I went through was purely mental, nothing

> physical, it was purely mental. To me that has a deeper aspect of creating a mental happiness and contentment. It's not dependent on material circumstances. (Charles, aged 50)

Charles's search for a spiritual *home* is connected to his personal history. The idea of a home resonates with feelings of attachment, security and relationship. By contrast, the principal difficulties of Charles's life were emotional loss, leading to a concern with 'mental happiness and contentment' more than with material possessions. In particular, his family 'home' involved a relationship with an alcoholic father that 'was distant and became troublesome. I became very angry with him'.

Charles felt that his family provided physical security but not love. 'I was basically unhappy,' he said. For many years, social isolation plagued his life: 'I've always found it difficult to make friends at school; I never fitted in at school.' He did enjoy college life more 'because there were a lot of deadbeats like me'. However, relationships were few and far between: 'I have always been very shy and socially I never quite learnt to fit in.' In a spiritual home, Charles belongs and he has friends.

Echoing the Buddhist concept of karma, Charles reflected on the fact that, while the past was gone, the present moment was built upon it. Karma contains the idea that what we do today has consequences for tomorrow; this is because of that. At 50, Charles was no longer the person who suffered as a 16-year-old. However, 'there's someone sitting here whose consciousness is partially dependent upon that experience'. He described this process as an 'evolution of consciousness' in which he had acquired greater levels of equanimity.

Equanimity is one of the purposes of spiritual practice. It involves a radical acceptance of 'what is'; an even-handedness towards events achieved through an understanding of their causes and conditions. For Charles, equanimity entails composure and 'the ability to remain balanced without identifying with stuff that you don't actually need to identify with'. For example, he told me about a relationship with a woman that had become troubled (he was no longer a monk). He experienced 'the churning of emotions' in which 'I could see this really needy person kind of emerging out of the shadows and I just refused to identify with it. It's not that I don't have needs, it's just that I refuse to identify with them'.

FRANK: THE GIFT OF RECOVERY

The reduction of psychological suffering was also at the core of Frank's remarkable life. Through a combination of psychotherapy and spiritual practice, Frank had transformed a troubled life into one of greater acceptance, peace and contentment. Indeed, he now described his extreme levels of suffering as 'a gift', a word he used on eight occasions in one conversation.

> I just think every day is a gift now. I wouldn't be where I'm at today, with the understanding that I have, if those things hadn't happened and that's why I believe the book is written; we just live it. So it's a sense of, we learn from suffering, we don't learn from the good times. We appreciate the good times because they balance the suffering, but the true learning curves are the suffering. Now we are brought up not to like that, instead of owning it. I have just learnt that the more I own it, I just accept the fact that something shitty can happen today and if it does, I'll fix it. I won't let it get me any more. I won't suffer from a panic attack in a car park anymore. The level of anxiety could still be there, but it won't be as great as it used to be. So it's adopting that proactive approach to whatever happens on the day – I'm gonna, you just have to greet each day and take it on board. (Frank, aged 38)

The influence of spiritual thinking on Frank is evident in the way he talks about the transformation of suffering. Buddhism teaches that we must learn from difficulties and come to equanimity. Happiness is not so much about getting what we want as wanting what we've got. We might describe this process as 'letting go' of the things that make us suffer. In particular, meditation involves learning to experience emotional difficulties without acting them out. Frank says by learning from his suffering he has come to accept levels of anxiety that he might previously have found intolerable.

Acceptance is surely at the heart of the phrase 'the book is written'. The notion of 'owning' his emotional experiences is, however, a phrase derived from Western psychology. Indeed, Frank sought to integrate spiritual practices with psychotherapy. On the one hand: 'I guess where I've actually found the most peace is in Tibetan Buddhism,' he said. However, on the other hand: 'Where I learnt most about compassion was in a psychiatric hospital amongst the other patients.'

As a child, Frank was physically mistreated by his mother and sexually abused by her lover, a man who later became his stepfather. The sexual abuse started when he was 11 and continued until he was 20. It included being drugged from the age of 15. As a consequence, 'I learnt to dissociate at a very young age'. In its milder form, disassociation entails distracting ourselves from the present moment through daydreaming or endlessly recycling thoughts in our mind. In its more severe mode, it entails an emotional 'numbness' and detachment from other people. In Frank's case, disassociation was pushed to the extreme of generating complete personalities. He also experienced acute anxiety and depression, leading to substance abuse. Intense disassociation of this type is often associated with post-traumatic stress disorder.

> By the time I was 34, I was actually diagnosed with DID, dissociative identity disorder, where there were five main personalities and about 19 other fragments. In essence I now appreciate that as a sense of oneness; they were all my coping strategies. (Frank, aged 38)

Frank told me that his condition was a response to childhood abuse that enabled him to distance himself from the painful reality of his experience. He developed this strategy to the point where coping mechanisms became alternative personalities. A shift from one 'personality' to another was commonly triggered by factors in the environment: a noise, a smell, a word, or an image. On some occasions, he was able to 'will' a personality change.

At some levels, Frank was able to cope. Indeed, he successfully advanced through the managerial ranks of retail companies. However, his 'workaholic' career advancement was a mask for emotional suffering. Frank suffered severe bouts of depression and drug abuse. He made three suicide attempts, leading to lengthy periods of hospitalisation.

Frank's recovery involved a two-and-a-half-year process of personality integration that he described as a 'buddy-up system'. This procedure is best addressed in the language of psychiatry, which lies beyond the scope of this chapter. We focus instead on his use of Buddhism as a supportive practice. Frank's key therapist introduced him to Eastern psychology, which he read enthusiastically. He attended a practice centre across the road from the hospital and began to understand himself through spiritual concepts. He made connections between them and psychotherapy. 'You could say that Buddha was the first cognitive behavioural therapist ever,' he argued.

The comparison Frank draws between cognitive therapy and Buddhism is one that others have also made because both involve mindfully examining one's own thought processes. We explore mindfulness-based cognitive therapy later in the chapter. In any case, the combination of psychotherapy and meditation enabled Frank 'to head towards that sense of peace or spiritual awareness that we are at one with the universe'. Asked how much Buddhism had been a part of his recovery, Frank replied with a phrase he used on three occasions: 'It was meant to be. The book was written and I just turn a page each day.'

Eastern meditation meets Western science

The emotional life stories told by David and Frank could hardly be more different. For David, mindfulness meditation was simply part of a life devoted to emotional balance. For Frank, it was a life raft thrown to a drowning man, a shining light amidst extreme pain and suffering. But for both men it was an emotionally beneficial practice, and one for which there is a growing body of supportive scientific evidence.

MEDITATION AND THE BRAIN

Since 1987, the Dalai Lama has been engaged in a series of discussions exploring the common ground (and areas of dispute) between (Tibetan) Buddhism and Western science. Two conferences concentrated on emotion and prompted a series of illuminating experiments carried out by Richard Davidson of the University of Wisconsin.[7] Using sophisticated functional magnetic resonance imaging (fMRI) scans, Davidson monitored the brain activity of an experienced Buddhist monk (under the pseudonym of Lama Oser) as he underwent a series of meditation exercises.

Davidson had already established that people demonstrating a higher ratio of activity in the left prefrontal cortex exhibit happier, more joyful temperaments and recover more swiftly from emotional setbacks. By contrast, a higher ratio of activity in the right prefrontal cortex is associated with fear, anxiety and depression. Most people are located in the middle ground with 67 per cent of subjects being moderately happy and 33 per cent placed on the outer edges of the spectrum. However, activity in Lama Oser's left prefrontal cortex was 'off the chart' even when not meditating. This suggests that meditation may increase the kind of brain activity that makes us happy.

Perhaps Lama Oser was a particularly lucky and contented person because he was born with a genetically determined 'happy' temperament. However, subsequent work by Davidson demonstrated that meditation actually increases left-sided brain activity. For example, his study of biotech workers found that, after eight weeks of meditation, levels of left-brain activity had grown, along with happier moods. Contemporary evidence suggests that the brain's emotional responses can be altered through training that reinforces particular patterns of electrical circuitry. Meditation seems to act cumulatively to strengthen the parts of the brain that calm fear and give rise to happiness. Further scientific investigation is providing evidence that meditation and mindfulness offer tangible benefits to mental health and emotional management.

MINDFULNESS AND MEDICINE

John Kabat-Zinn[8] pioneered the practices of mindfulness within Western medicine at the University of Massachusetts' Stress Reduction Clinic. He deployed them in the treatment of heart disease, anxiety, panic attack and chronic pain. He demonstrated that patients experienced long-lasting physical and psychological benefits from meditation. Kabat-Zinn's work is primarily concerned with the psychological components of physical illness. But Western psychology has also become interested in the value of mindfulness in the management of emotional distress.

Some practitioners of cognitive therapy have appropriated mindfulness to treat depression, anxiety and borderline personality disorder.

Cognitive therapy is founded on the idea that recurrent negative thoughts of loss, failure, worthlessness and rejection are not simply symptoms of depression but causes. Patients are therefore encouraged to monitor their thoughts in order to examine them for their usefulness and veracity. Studies confirm the efficacy of cognitive therapy in the treatment of depression.[9] Mindfulness entails paying attention to the present moment, and so like cognitive therapy we observe the flow of thinking. There is now evidence that meditation and mindfulness can play an effective part in the treatment of depression.

MINDFULNESS-BASED COGNITIVE THERAPY FOR DEPRESSION

Segal, Williams and Teasdale[10] developed mindfulness-based cognitive therapy for depression (MBCT) and presented evidence that it reduces relapse rates. They proposed a learnt association between mood and patterns of thinking by which a sad feeling, however induced, reactivates the mindset associated with previous depression-inducing moods. A person with a history of depression is thus more likely (and with greater speed) to turn a sad mood into a more persistent and intense condition.

Depression is associated with a 'ruminative response style'. Sufferers go over and over incidents and feelings in a ceaseless cycle. This prolongs and deepens their unhappiness because it is part of the depression. To end the blue mood, it is necessary to break the constant cycle of chewing over thoughts. We need to develop space in the mind so that awareness can recognise thinking as 'just thoughts' rather than solidified reality.

Segal and his colleagues anticipated that 'mindfulness' would allow patients to notice when they are about to undergo perilous mood swings, enabling them to undercut the hazardous process of rumination. If patients could cease their relentless circular reflections, they would escape depression-linked thought patterns. It was hoped that mindfulness would allow people to leave behind constant attention to the perceived inadequacies of their lives.

Segal and his colleagues tested their ideas in an experiment involving 145 patients. They taught volunteers skills of mindfulness and compared them with a group who had not undergone this training. Their evidence suggests that for patients undergoing MBCT who had experienced three or more previous episodes of depression (77 per cent of the sample) relapse rates after five years were 37 per cent, compared to 66 per cent for patients receiving treatment as usual. However, MBCT was no more effective than 'treatment as usual' in patients with less than three previous depressive episodes. This may be because MBCT worked to disrupt automatic relapse mechanisms (particularly the rumination process) that become of greater significance with more frequent depressions.

JON AND STEVE: ORDINARY SUFFERING

Both Frank's extreme misery and David's contentment were unusual emotional states among the men I spoke with. Mostly, these meditators thought themselves confronted with the ordinary suffering of the human condition. Jon was not abused as a child and hailed from a family that we would normally see as 'good enough'. Yet, he felt isolated and lacking in the loving relationships he desired. He talked about loneliness and a 'feeling of grief around not being loved. There was a feeling of pain around not having the feeling of a real kind of emotional connectedness with either of my parents' (Jon, aged 40).

Jon felt that his experience of family life was no different from other people's, but of course emotional distress is not dependent on suffering the severe trauma of Frank's life. Routine emotional neglect is quite enough for normal unhappiness.

> I kind of reconnected into Buddhist stuff and meditation again, into exploring myself a bit more actively, you know, not having any choice really but to deal with psychological issues and stuff that I needed to process and examine, you know, to shine a light on. (Jon, aged 40)

Jon's 'reconnection' with Buddhism was a long and winding road through hippie communes, religious cults, drug use, travel to Asia and bouts of depression. Like most of these men, his adoption of spiritual practices was a developmental process. The metaphor 'to shine a light on' is a classic Buddhist phrase that chimes with the mythical last words of the Buddha that one should 'be a lamp unto oneself'. The phrase suggests that we need to explore our own thoughts, feelings, motivations and actions in order to discover the sources of our suffering, and that it is our responsibility to do so. We are invited to shine the lamp of mindfulness upon ourselves. The main feature of Jon's life on which he needed to shine that light was 'relationship dramas and relationship pain': the end of relationships, the experience of emotional aloneness.

Like Jon, Steve (aged 42) did not experience anything that our culture would normally understand as abuse. However, within his childhood family lie the roots of a melancholy personality prone to self-criticism and moderate depression: 'I had pretty loving parents, but there was an underlying criticalness.' Steve became 'a bit of a loner' and felt that 'I have a bit of a problem around intimacy, which is a bit of a men's issue, I guess'. He continued: 'The Zen thing gave me a kind of stability and actually one of the other things I think that it did for me was to start to give me a way of connecting with people.' Above all, mindfulness helped Steve to 'face reality' and 'be able to tolerate the way things are and not trying to make it perfect'.

A grounded spirituality

Freed from the irrationalities of medieval religion, contemporary spirituality is concerned with meaning and emotional balance. It is sceptical and does not require superstitious beliefs or blind faith. This grounded spirituality is self-reflective and plays a necessary part in the emotional lives of human beings. Though our white-bearded supernatural God has died, we human beings still need purpose, ethics and love. It's in our genes.

Of course, neither meaning nor emotional balance is confined to the obviously 'spiritual'. On the face of it, football does not have much in common with spirituality, but as we noted in chapter 2, the emotional wellbeing of sportsmen owes much to their constructive thinking, sense of purpose and extensive friendship network. Sport and spirituality at their best are characterised by good habits developed through training and self-discipline. In their different ways, they are both pragmatic and grounded practices of self-transformation.

For David, contemporary spirituality provides:

> A perspective, a confidence, an awareness within which one can embrace and count one's experience. A sense of knowing who one is and what one isn't. A sense of feeling connected to humanity and even beyond humanity; a connectedness to nature, to beingness; being able to put things in a much broader perspective of life and of lives rather than being just caught up in the small-minded pettiness of mundane issues. Being able to focus attention on mundane issues, but at the same time when it's appropriate, being able to fall back into the bigger perspective of, okay, this will pass; in the great scheme of things it's not that important. Being able to feel more connected to the essence of being a human being or in touch with feelings, emotions, more aware of desires and aversions. (David, aged 37)

David's explanation of spirituality ties together the themes of this chapter and indeed the whole book. For him, it concerns our *awareness* of *experience* in ways that *connect* us with all life and put our own existence into a meaningful *broader perspective*. Spirituality involves learning to *focus attention* on the *mundane* as a part of a *bigger perspective*, knowing that all things are impermanent and *will pass*. In this way, we are able to be more aware of the nature of our *emotions*.

I have no doubt that my engagement with mindfulness meditation as presented by Thich Nhat Hanh played a part in my recovery from depression. I learnt to tell myself repeatedly that depression would pass; all things are impermanent. More generally, I have learnt to pay greater attention to what I am thinking and doing. For example, as I walk from the car park to my office at work, I pass by a small stream. The gentle sound reminds me to stop, listen and still my mind. Then I walk on slowly and arrive at my desk in a much calmer condition than I once did. It is important to try to do things more slowly.

The practices of mindfulness have helped me to reduce anxiety, remain calm and maintain a greater emotional balance. I have developed a stronger sense of an awareness that is not identified with the stream of language. This has assisted me to reduce that rumination which fuels depressed moods and to sit through difficult feelings rather than act them out. I also pay more attention to the wonders of life. It is important to develop gratitude for the good things and not to focus only on difficulties. Research has shown that people who increase gratitude maintain more positive moods, are more alert, and have fewer physical ailments.[11]

I have also been reminded to cultivate relationships with other people and once again seek an ethical basis for the pursuit of justice. As a young man, I had been politically active on the 'left', but as I got older I not only lost a degree of practical commitment but also any conviction in the available theories of emancipation (for example, Marxism). Buddhism has restored my ethical purpose and the possibility of personal and social change. I am not trying to claim enlightenment (whatever that is) or to suggest that mindfulness meditation has solved all my problems. But I am much more content, and when difficulties arise I now have better ways to restore myself.

On reflection

THE QUALITY OF LOVE

Our personal lives are intertwined with the social world, and so throughout this book I have explored men's emotions as cultural stories. These narratives demonstrate that men can and do speak about emotion. This is not to say that when men speak about emotion they are necessarily skilful (but neither are women). In particular, we encountered a powerful stream of men struggling with depression, alcohol/drug abuse and poor relationships because of the way they think. We also witnessed a range of more productive strategies associated with happier men.

An understanding of the emotional lives of men must acknowledge the key social changes that are impacting them; that is, the restructuring of work, family and relationships. Nonetheless, the central pattern of men's individual emotional strategies derives from attachment processes in childhood families. I am not suggesting that there is only one desirable family form. I am not arguing for a return to conservative family values. But I am pointing to the *ethic of love* as being critical to the wellbeing of individuals and cultures.

Our culture's emphasis on individualism and material wealth in the context of global uncertainty is amplifying emotional difficulties. Because of our attachment to work and individual achievement, men are particularly prone to self-absorption and social isolation. Of course, we can't simply turn the historical clock back even if we wanted to, which we probably don't. However, we can adopt outlooks, policies and practices that strengthen human love, co-operation and solidarity. Our emotional wellbeing depends on developing the quality of our relationships.

TOWARDS HAPPINESS

Western psychology and Eastern spiritual traditions are both concerned with the causes of emotional suffering and the conditions of happiness. They share a focus on the skilful management of difficult emotions, including anger, anxiety and depression; as well as the promotion of contentment. Both suggest that wealth is not the key to a happy life. Rather, joy and depression are founded in our attitudes, beliefs and actions. Love, compassion and emotional balance are all vital to happiness and these are qualities that we can develop. We can reduce despair and increase happiness by changing the way we think and behave. But we do have to work at it.

And this concern with individual wellbeing need not be just another Western obsession with the self. On the one hand, individuals can only be happy in a social context. The sense of purpose each of us needs must be achieved within a wider community ethics of the good and meaningful life. But also, personal strategies have social implications. Happy men contribute to peaceful societies; angry despairing men bring violence and misery to those around them. When I look after myself, I care for others; when I care for others, I look after myself.

Notes

Chapter 1   Stories of modern men

1. Stephen had been diagnosed as suffering from attention deficit disorder as a child.
2. I conducted 107 interviews, all of which informed the argument of the book. The words of more than 80 men are directly quoted in the book. All names have been changed.
3. It can be assumed for the remainder of the book that I am discussing modern Western culture and that conclusions cannot necessarily be applied to other cultures.
4. Stearns, PN & Knapp, M (1996) 'Historical perspectives on grief', in R Harre and WG Parrott (eds) *The Emotions: Social, Cultural and Biological Dimensions*. London: Sage.
5. Cohen, S (1972) *Folk Devils and Moral Panics: The Creation of the Mods and Rockers*. London: MacGibbon & Kee.
6. Real, T (1998) *I Don't Want to Talk About It: Men and Depression*. Dublin: Newleaf.
7. These 'story' sections are entirely made up of the men's words, though I have edited them to make them more compact and fluent.
8. Farrell, W (1993) *The Myth of Male Power*. Sydney: Random House.
9. Two professional basketball players, a professional basketball coach, three professional rugby players (one rugby league and two rugby union), a professional rugby coach, a professional cricketer, a pro-golfer and a former Olympic athlete turned professional coach.
10. Two Australian Rules football players, two surfers, two athletes, two soccer players, two rugby players and a hockey player.

Chapter 2 This sporting life

1. Lineham, M (1993) *Cognitive-Behavioural Treatment for Borderline Personality Disorder*. New York: The Guilford Press.
2. Connell, R (1990) 'An iron man: The body and some contradictions of hegemonic masculinity', in MA Messner & DF Sabo (eds) *Sport, Men, and the Gender Order: Critical Feminist Perspectives*. Champaign, IL: Human Kinetics; Sabo, DF (1994) 'Pigskin, patriarchy and pain', in MA Messner & DF Sabo *Sex, Violence and Power in Sport: Rethinking Masculinity*. Freedom, CA: Crossing Press.
3. Hamilton, M (2006) *What Men Don't Talk About*. Sydney: Viking Penguin.
4. Foucault, M (1977) *Discipline and Punishment*. London: Allen Lane.
5. Foucault, M (1986) *The Care of the Self: The History of Sexuality*, vol. 3. London: Penguin.
6. Seligman, M (2002) *Authentic Happiness*. Sydney: Random House.

Chapter 3 Why we are talking about men now

1. LeDoux, J (1998) *The Emotional Brain*. London: Phoenix.
2. Real, T (1998) *I Don't Want to Talk About It: Men and Depression*. Dublin: Newleaf.
3. Biddulph, S (1994) *Manhood*. Sydney: Finch.
4. Claire, A (2000) *On Men: Masculinity in Crisis*. London: Chatto & Windus.
5. Farrell, W (1993) *The Myth of Male Power*. Sydney: Random House.
6. In addition to Biddulph, Claire and Real above, see also: Connell, RW (1995) *Masculinities*. Cambridge: Polity Press; Faludi, S (1999) *Stiffed: The Betrayal of the American Man*. London: Chatto & Windus; Giddens, A (1992) *The Transformation of Intimacy*. Cambridge: Polity Press; Lee, J (1991) *At My Fathers Wedding*. New York: Bantam Books; Lupton, D (1998) *The Emotional Self*. London: Sage; Kimmel, MS, Hearn, J & Connell, RW (eds) (2005) *Handbook of Studies on Men and Masculinities*. London & Thousand Oaks: Sage.
7. Faludi, S (1999) *Stiffed: The Betrayal of the American Man*. London: Chatto & Windus.
8. Faludi (1999), p. 30.
9. Claire, A (2000) *On Men: Masculinity in Crisis*. London: Chatto & Windus.
10. Stacey, J (1996) *In the Name of the Family: Rethinking Family Values in a Postmodern World*. Boston: Beacon Press.
11. Giddens, A (1992) *The Transformation of Intimacy*. Cambridge: Polity Press.

Chapter 4 Your mum and dad

1. Deveson, A (2003) *Resilience*. Sydney: Allen & Unwin.
2. Real, T (1998) *I Don't Want to Talk About It: Men and Depression*. Dublin: Newleaf.

3   See Faludi, S (1999) *Stiffed: The Betrayal of the American Man*. London: Chatto & Windus, for a sympathetic sociological approach from a feminist writer and Real, above, for a psychologically oriented view. See Biddulph, S (1994) *Manhood*. Sydney: Finch; Bly, R (1991) *Iron John: A Book About Men*. London: Element; and Lee, J (1991) *At My Fathers Wedding*. New York: Bantam Books, for 'mythopoetic' men's movement perspectives. An interesting novel connected to the theme is O'Hagen, A (1999) *Our Fathers*. London: Faber & Faber.
4   Hite, S (1994) *The Hite Report on the Family*. London: Bloomsbury.
5   See Nussbaum, M (2002) *Upheavals of Thought: The Intelligence of Emotion*. Cambridge: Cambridge University Press, for a review of these issues.
6   Young JE & Klosko, JS (1993) *Reinventing Your Life*. New York: Plume.

Chapter 5   Family foundations

1   Chodorow, N (1978) *The Reproduction of Motherhood*. Berkeley: University of California Press; Giddens, A (1992) *The Transformation of Intimacy*. Cambridge: Polity Press.
2   Goleman, D (1995) *Emotional Intelligence*. New York: Bantam Books.
3   Nussbaum, M (2002) *Upheavals of Thought: The Intelligence of Emotion*. Cambridge: Cambridge University Press.
4   Seligman, M (1990) *Learned Optimism*. Sydney: Random House.
5   Bowlby, J (1980) *Attachment and Loss*. London: Hogarth Press.
6   Herman, J (1992) *Trauma and Recovery*. New York: Basic Books.
7   Crowell, JA & Treboux, D (1995) 'A review of adult attachment measures: Implications for theory and research'. *Social Development*, 4: 294–377. All subsequent references to research in this chapter refer to this paper.
8   Crowell & Treboux (1995).
9   Young, JE & Klosko, JS (1993) *Reinventing Your Life*. New York: Plume.

Chapter 6   Men and depression

1   These figures were taken on 25 September 2006 from the following websites:
    <http://www.upliftprogram.com>
    <http://www.beyondblue.org.au>
    <http://www.depressionnet.com.au>
2   Lepine, JP, Gastpar, M, Mendlewicz, J & Tylee, A (1997) 'Depression in the community: The first pan-European study DEPRES'. *International Clinical Psychopharmacology*, 12: 12–29.
3   Segal, Z, Williams, J & Teasdale, J (2002) *Mindfulness-Based Cognitive Therapy for Depression: A New Approach to Preventing Relapse*. New York and London: The Guilford Press.
4   <http://www.abs.gov.au>.
5   <http://www.depressionnet.com.au.newsletter/nl-stats.html>.
6   Hassan, R (1997) 'Suicide trends in Australia', in K Healey (ed.) *Suicide*, vol. 84. Sydney: The Spinney Press.

7   Lennane, J (1997) 'Youth suicide: Why us?', in K Healey (ed.) *Suicide*, vol. 84. Sydney: The Spinney Press.
8   <http://www.beyondblue.org.au>.
9   Rowe, D (1996) *Depression: The Way Out of Your Prison*. London: Routledge, p. 3.
10 Adapted from Tanner, S & Ball, J (1991) *Beating the Blues*. Sydney: Tanner/Ball.
11 Hamer, D & Copeland, P (1998) *Living with Our Genes*. New York: Doubleday.
12 Sloman, L (2000) 'The syndrome of rejection sensitivity: An evolutionary perspective', in Gilbert, P and Baily, K *Genes on the Couch: Explorations in Evolutionary Psychotherapy*. Hove: Brunner-Routledge.
13 Herman, J (1992) *Trauma and Recovery*. New York: Basic Books.
14 Aron, E (2003) *The Highly Sensitive Person*. London: HarperCollins.
15 Seligman, M (1990) *Learned Optimism*. Sydney: Random House.

Chapter 7   Living on drugs and alcohol

1   Giddens, A (1992) *The Transformation of Intimacy*. Cambridge: Polity Press.
2   Giddens (1992), p. 76.
3   Vanzant, I (2000) 'When you feel ...', *Until Today*. New York: Simon & Schuster.

Chapter 8   Work, work, work

1   Elias, N (1978) *The History of Manners: The Civilizing Process*, vol. 1. Oxford: Blackwell.
2   Giddens, A (1992) *The Transformation of Intimacy*. Cambridge: Polity Press.
3   *The Sydney Morning Herald*, 5–6 February 2005.
4   Shumaker, J (2001) *The Age of Insanity: Modernity and Mental Health*. Westport: Praeger.

Chapter 9   Men and relationships

1   Seligman, M (2002). *Authentic Happiness*. Sydney: Random House.
2   Claire, A (2000) *On Men: Masculinity in Crisis*. London: Chatto & Windus.
3   Fitness, J (2001) 'Emotional intelligence and intimate relationships', in Ciarrochi, J, Forgas, J & Mayer, J (eds) *Emotional Intelligence in Everyday Life*. Philadelphia and Hove: Taylor & Francis.
4   Giddens, A (1992) *The Transformation of Intimacy*. Cambridge: Polity Press.
5   Schnarch, D (1999) *Passionate Marriage: Keeping Love and Intimacy Alive in Committed Relationships*. Carlton: Scribe Publications.
6   Duncombe, J & Marsden, D (1993) 'Love and intimacy: The gender division of emotion and emotion work' *Sociology*, 27: 221–41.
7   See *The Sydney Morning Herald*, 5–6 February 2005.
8   Relationships Australia (2003) *Relationships Indicators Survey 2003*. At: <http://www.relationships.com.au/utilities/about/stats.asp>.
9   de Vaus, P (2004) *Diversity and Change in Australian Families*. Melbourne: Australian Institute of Family Studies.

Chapter 10 Changing ourselves

1. Lineham, M (1993) *Cognitive-Behavioural Treatment for Borderline Personality Disorder*. New York: The Guilford Press; Lineham, M (1993) *Skills Training Manual for Treating Borderline Personality Disorder*. London and New York: The Guilford Press.
2. Prochaska, J, Norcross, J & DiClemente, C (1994) *Changing for Good*. New York: William Morrow.
3. Seligman, M (2002) *Authentic Happiness*. Sydney: Random House.
4. Seligman (2002), p. 262.
5. Seligman (2002), p. 263.
6. Thich Nhat Hanh (2001) *Transformation at the Base*. Berkeley, CA: Parallax Press.

Chapter 11 Redemption song

1. Zohar, D & Marshall, I (2000) *SQ Spiritual Intelligence: The Ultimate Intelligence*. London: Bloomsbury, p. 4.
2. Giddens, A (1991) *Modernity and Self-Identity*. Cambridge: Polity Press.
3. Tacey, D (2003) *The Spirituality Revolution*. Sydney: HarperCollins; Young-Eisendrath, P & Miller, M (2000) 'Beyond enlightened self-interest: The psychology of mature spirituality in the twenty-first century', in P Young-Eisendrath & M Miller (eds) *The Psychology of Mature Spirituality*. London: Routledge.
4. Thich Nhat Hanh (1975) *The Miracle of Mindfulness*. Berkeley, CA: Parallax Press, p. 7.
5. Thich Naht Hahn (1990) *Present Moment, Wonderful Moment*. Berkeley, CA: Parallax Press.
6. Dharma here means Buddhist teachings and practices.
7. Goleman, D (2003) *Destructive Emotions and How We Can Overcome Them: A Dialogue with The Dalai Lama*. London: Bloomsbury.
8. Kabat-Zinn, J (1990) *Full Catastrophe Living: Using the Wisdom of Your Body and Mind to Face Stress, Pain, and Illness*. New York: Delta.
9. Segal, Z, Williams, J & Teasdale, J (2002) *Mindfulness-Based Cognitive Therapy for Depression: A New Approach to Preventing Relapse*. New York and London: The Guilford Press.
10. Segal, Williams & Teasdale (2002).
11. Emmons, RA & McCullough, ME (2003) 'Counting blessings versus burdens: Experimental studies of gratitude and subjective well-being in daily life'. *Journal of Personality and Social Psychology*, 84: 377–89.